Prologue

The first gentle flutter of life inside Sarah was barely perceptible, like a soft whisper that barely disturbed the surface of her thoughts. It was a quiet evening in early spring, the kind when the world seems to pause, holding its breath before the onset of new life. Sarah was curled up on the sofa, a knitted blanket draped over her legs, her mind a mix of anticipation and fatigue from the whirlwind of the past few months.

As she sat in the dim light of their cozy living room, the realization of what she had felt began to settle in. The sensation was fleeting and delicate, a subtle reminder that their long-held dream was becoming a reality. She placed her hand gently over her abdomen, feeling a tender connection that seemed to bridge the gap between their hopes and the unfolding reality.

Jake's work had been demanding lately, and the house had been unusually quiet in his absence. The evenings were often filled with Sarah's solitary thoughts and the gentle ticking of the old clock on the wall. But tonight was different. Tonight, the quiet was filled with a promise of new beginnings.

Sarah's heart raced as she thought about how to share this miraculous moment with Jake. Their journey to this point had been a delicate dance of hope and patience, a series of highs and lows that had tested their resolve. They had faced uncertainty and heartache, yet their dreams of expanding their family had remained a beacon of light guiding them through the darkest moments.

With a deep breath, Sarah picked up her phone and dialed Jake's number. The anticipation made her hands tremble slightly as she waited for him to answer. When his voice came through, warm and familiar, she felt a rush of relief and excitement.

"Hey, Sarah. Everything okay?" Jake's voice was tinged with concern.

"I need you to come home," Sarah said, her voice trembling with emotion. "I felt something. I think…it's our baby."

Jake's silence was a mix of surprise and curiosity. "I'm on my way."

As she waited for him, Sarah looked around their living room, the familiar surroundings now feeling charged with the promise of change. The room, with its comfortable furniture and the soft glow of the lamp, seemed to be holding its breath, sharing in her anticipation.

When Jake finally arrived, his expression shifted from weariness to wonder as Sarah took his hand and guided him to the sofa. She placed his hand gently on her abdomen, her eyes locked with his, searching for the same sense of awe she felt.

"Is it really happening?" Jake asked, his voice a soft whisper.

Sarah nodded, tears of joy welling in her eyes. "I felt a flutter. I think we're going to have a baby."

The moment hung between them, filled with the quiet excitement of a new beginning. As they embraced, the world outside seemed to blur, leaving only the two of them and the tiny, miraculous life growing within Sarah.

In that precious, quiet moment, they stood on the cusp of a journey that would transform their lives forever. With hearts full of hope and eyes turned toward the future, they were ready to welcome the new chapter that lay ahead, a chapter marked by the heartbeat of their dreams coming true.

Chapter 1: The Unexpected News

Sarah Matthews woke up to the sound of her alarm clock, its incessant beeping cutting through the remnants of her sleep. She reached over to silence it, groaning softly as she did. The morning light filtered through the curtains, casting a soft glow around the room. She lay there for a moment, gathering the energy to start her day. It was a Tuesday, and she had a full schedule at work. As a marketing manager for a rising tech firm, her days were often packed with meetings, presentations, and deadlines. But today, something felt different.

As Sarah got out of bed and made her way to the bathroom, she felt a wave of nausea wash over her. She paused, gripping the edge of the sink for support. This wasn't the first time she'd felt queasy recently, but she had chalked it up to stress and fatigue. Still, she couldn't ignore the nagging feeling that something else might be going on. Pushing the thought aside, she splashed her face with cold water and proceeded with her morning routine.

By the time she reached the kitchen, Jake, her fiancé, was already there, sipping his coffee and scrolling through his phone. He looked up and smiled as she entered the room.

"Morning, babe," he said, setting his mug down and walking over to give her a quick kiss. "You look pale. Everything okay?"

Sarah forced a smile. "Just tired, I guess. Didn't sleep well last night."

Jake frowned, concern etching his features. "You've been saying that a lot lately. Maybe you should see a doctor, just to be sure it's nothing serious."

She nodded absentmindedly, reaching for the kettle to make herself some tea. "Yeah, maybe. I'll think about it."

As the day wore on, Sarah's discomfort grew. At work, she found it hard to concentrate, her mind drifting back to the persistent nausea and fatigue she had been experiencing. During a particularly dull meeting, she found herself daydreaming, her thoughts wandering to the possibility of pregnancy. Could that be it? She and Jake had talked about starting a family someday, but they hadn't been actively trying. Still, accidents happen.

By lunchtime, Sarah couldn't take it anymore. She excused herself from a team meeting, telling her colleagues she wasn't feeling well. She drove to the nearest pharmacy and bought a pregnancy test, her heart pounding in her chest. She felt a mix of excitement and dread as she made her way back to the office, the small box burning a hole in her purse.

Unable to wait until she got home, Sarah locked herself in the office bathroom and took the test. The few minutes it took for the result to appear felt like an eternity. She stared at the little window, her breath catching in her throat as she saw the two pink lines. Positive. She was pregnant.

Sarah sat down on the toilet seat, the test still in her hand. She felt a rush of emotions: shock, disbelief, fear, and, surprisingly, a flicker of joy. She hadn't expected this, but as the reality sank in, she realized that part of her was already thinking about the future, about the tiny life growing inside her.

Her thoughts were interrupted by a knock on the bathroom door. "Sarah? Are you okay in there?" It was Emily, her coworker and friend.

Sarah quickly composed herself, shoving the test back into its box and into her purse. "Yeah, I'm fine," she called out, trying to keep her voice steady. "Just needed a moment."

When she finally emerged, Emily gave her a concerned look. "You sure you're okay? You've been looking a bit off all day."

Sarah forced a smile. "I'm fine, really. Just feeling a bit under the weather. I think I might head home early."

Emily nodded, still looking worried. "Alright. Take care of yourself, okay?"

Sarah gathered her things and left the office, her mind racing. She needed to talk to Jake, but how would she tell him? They had always been open with each other, but this was big. She didn't want to spring it on him over dinner like it was just another piece of news.

The drive home felt surreal. She kept glancing at her reflection in the rearview mirror, wondering if she looked different, if she looked like someone who was about to become a mother. By the time she pulled into the driveway, she had decided to tell Jake as soon as he got home from work.

Sarah spent the rest of the afternoon pacing the house, trying to keep herself busy. She tidied up, cooked dinner, and tried to distract herself with a book, but her mind kept drifting back to the test. Finally, she heard Jake's car pull into the driveway. Her heart began to race again.

Jake walked in, setting his briefcase by the door and kicking off his shoes. "Hey, honey. How was your day?"

Sarah took a deep breath, trying to steady her nerves. "It was…eventful. We need to talk."

Jake's brow furrowed in concern. "What's wrong? Are you feeling okay?"

She nodded, taking his hand and leading him to the couch. "I'm fine. But there's something I need to tell you."

Jake sat down, his eyes never leaving hers. "Okay. What is it?"

Sarah took a deep breath, the words catching in her throat. "I'm pregnant."

For a moment, there was silence. Jake stared at her, his expression unreadable. Then, slowly, a smile spread across his face. "You're pregnant?"

he repeated, as if trying to make sure he had heard her correctly.

She nodded, tears welling up in her eyes. "Yes. I took a test today, and it was positive."

Jake let out a breath he hadn't realized he was holding and pulled her into his arms. "That's amazing," he said, his voice filled with emotion. "I mean, it's unexpected, but…amazing."

Sarah felt a wave of relief wash over her as she hugged him back. She had been so worried about his reaction, but now that she was in his arms, she knew they would face this together. They had always been a team, and this was just another challenge they would conquer side by side.

Over the next few days, Sarah and Jake talked about their future, their hopes, and their fears. They knew that their lives were about to change in ways they couldn't even imagine, but they were ready to face it together. They started to make plans, talking about baby names, nursery ideas, and how they would balance their careers with parenthood.

Sarah also made an appointment with her doctor to confirm the pregnancy and to start prenatal care. As she sat in the waiting room, she felt a mixture of excitement and nervousness. This was really happening. She was going to be a mother.

The doctor confirmed the pregnancy, and as Sarah listened to the sound of her baby's heartbeat for the first time, she felt a profound sense of awe. There was a tiny life growing inside her, a life that she and Jake had created together. It was a feeling unlike anything she had ever experienced.

As the weeks went by, Sarah began to experience the early symptoms of pregnancy in full force. Morning sickness, fatigue, and mood swings became part of her daily routine. But despite the discomfort, she found herself growing more and more excited about the future. She and Jake attended their first prenatal class, where they learned about what to expect in the coming months. They met other expectant parents and began to build a support network.

Sarah's friends and family were thrilled when she shared the news. Her parents were especially excited about becoming grandparents. They offered advice and support, and Sarah appreciated their enthusiasm, even if it was a bit overwhelming at times.

One evening, as Sarah and Jake sat on the couch looking through baby name books, she turned to him and said, "Can you believe we're going to be parents?"

Jake smiled, squeezing her hand. "It's a little scary, but I'm so excited. We're going to be great parents, Sarah. I just know it."

Sarah rested her head on his shoulder, feeling a sense of contentment wash over her. They still had a long journey ahead, but for the first time in a long while, she felt like everything was going to be okay.

As the first trimester progressed, Sarah and Jake continued to prepare for their new arrival. They started to buy baby clothes and furniture, transforming the spare bedroom into a nursery. They spent weekends assembling cribs and painting walls, each task bringing them closer together.

Sarah also began to take better care of herself, focusing on eating healthy and staying active. She joined a prenatal yoga class, which helped her relax and connect with other expectant mothers. The support she found in the class was invaluable, and she made several new friends who were going through the same experiences.

Despite the challenges and the occasional bouts of anxiety, Sarah found herself embracing her pregnancy. She marveled at the changes in her body, the way her belly grew and the way she could feel her baby move inside her. Each flutter and kick was a reminder of the new life she was nurturing.

One evening, as Sarah and Jake sat on the couch, she felt a strong kick. She grabbed Jake's hand and placed it on her belly. "Feel that?"

Jake's eyes widened as he felt the movement. "Wow, that's incredible. Our baby is really in there."

Sarah smiled, tears of joy in her eyes. "Yes, our baby. I can't wait to meet them."

As the weeks turned into months, Sarah and Jake grew more excited about the future. They knew that there would be challenges ahead, but they were ready to face them together. They were ready to become a family.

In the end, the unexpected news had turned into the most wonderful surprise of their lives. Sarah knew that the journey ahead would be filled with ups and downs, but she also knew that she had Jake by her side, and that made all the difference. As she looked forward to the future, she felt a sense of peace and happiness that she had never known before. She was ready for whatever came next, and she knew that she and Jake would face it together, one step at a time.

Chapter 2: Sharing the News

The days following Sarah's discovery of her pregnancy were a whirlwind of emotions. She and Jake spent countless hours talking, planning, and dreaming about their future. The initial shock had given way to a deep sense of excitement, but there was still a lingering anxiety about how their families and friends would react to the news.

One evening, as they sat on the couch, Sarah looked at Jake, her eyes filled with a mix of excitement and apprehension. "We need to start telling people," she said, her voice barely above a whisper.

Jake nodded, understanding the weight of her words. "Yeah, we do. Have you thought about how you want to do it?"

Sarah bit her lip, considering her options. "I think we should start with our parents. They deserve to know first."

Jake agreed. "Absolutely. Do you want to tell them together or separately?"

"Together," Sarah said firmly. "It feels right to do it as a team."

The following weekend, they invited Sarah's parents, David and Linda, over for dinner. As Sarah prepared the meal, her mind raced with thoughts of how they would react. Her parents had always been supportive, but this was big news.

Jake could sense her nervousness and came up behind her, wrapping his arms around her waist. "It's going to be fine," he murmured, kissing her temple. "They're going to be thrilled."

"I hope so," Sarah replied, leaning into his embrace. "I just want everything to go smoothly."

When her parents arrived, the house was filled with the aroma of roast chicken and fresh vegetables. They exchanged hugs and pleasantries, and Sarah tried to keep her nerves in check as they sat down to dinner.

As they ate, the conversation flowed naturally, but Sarah could feel the weight of the unspoken news hanging over them. Finally, as they were finishing dessert, Jake gave her a reassuring nod.

"Mom, Dad, there's something we need to tell you," Sarah began, her heart pounding in her chest.

David and Linda exchanged curious glances, setting down their forks. "What is it, sweetheart?" David asked, his voice gentle.

Sarah took a deep breath, reaching for Jake's hand. "We're going to have a baby."

For a moment, there was silence. Then, Linda's eyes filled with tears of joy. "Oh, Sarah, that's wonderful news!" she exclaimed, reaching across the table to take her daughter's hand.

David's face broke into a broad smile. "Congratulations, you two. This is incredible. We're so happy for you."

Sarah felt a wave of relief wash over her as her parents stood up to hug her and Jake. Their joy was palpable, and it reassured her that everything was going to be alright.

They spent the rest of the evening discussing the pregnancy, sharing their hopes and dreams for the future. Linda offered to help with the nursery, while David shared stories of when Sarah was a baby. It was a night filled with love and laughter, and by the time her parents left, Sarah felt a deep sense of contentment.

The next step was telling Jake's parents. They decided to visit them the following weekend. Jake's parents, Robert and Karen, lived a few hours away, so they planned a day trip. As they drove, Sarah couldn't help but feel a bit anxious again. She had always gotten along well with Jake's parents, but she knew that big news like this could be unpredictable.

When they arrived, Robert and Karen greeted them warmly, inviting them in for coffee. They sat in the cozy living room, chatting about the latest family news and local events.

Finally, Jake cleared his throat, glancing at Sarah. "Mom, Dad, there's something we want to share with you."

Karen looked at them expectantly. "What is it, dear?"

Jake smiled, squeezing Sarah's hand. "We're going to have a baby."

Karen gasped, her eyes lighting up with excitement. "Oh my goodness, that's amazing news!" she exclaimed, standing up to hug them both.

Robert's face broke into a proud grin. "Congratulations! We're so happy for you."

They spent the rest of the day talking about the baby, sharing their excitement and plans. Karen offered to knit some baby clothes, while Robert promised to build a crib. By the time they left, Sarah felt a renewed sense of joy and anticipation.

With their parents informed, it was time to tell their friends. Sarah and Jake decided to host a small gathering at their house, inviting their closest friends for a casual barbecue. They wanted to share the news in a relaxed and joyful setting.

As the day of the barbecue approached, Sarah felt a mix of excitement and nerves. She and Jake spent the morning preparing, setting up the backyard and grilling food. Their friends arrived in the early afternoon, bringing laughter and warmth to their home.

After everyone had eaten and was lounging around the backyard, Jake stood up, tapping his glass to get everyone's attention. "Hey, everyone, can we have your attention for a moment?"

The group fell silent, turning to look at them expectantly. Sarah felt her heart race as she stood beside Jake, her hand in his.

"We have some news to share," Jake continued, glancing at Sarah. "Sarah and I are expecting a baby."

The response was immediate and overwhelming. Their friends erupted in cheers and congratulations, rushing over to hug them and offer their well-wishes. Sarah felt tears of joy prick her eyes as she was enveloped in the warmth and love of her friends.

As the evening went on, the conversation was filled with excitement about the baby. Sarah's friend Emily, who had suspected something was up, gave her a knowing smile. "I had a feeling," she said, hugging Sarah tightly. "I'm so happy for you."

The rest of the evening was a blur of joy and celebration. Sarah felt incredibly grateful for the support and love of their friends. It was a reminder that they were not alone on this journey.

As the weeks went by, Sarah and Jake continued to share the news with more family members and friends. Each announcement was met with excitement and congratulations, and they felt their support network growing stronger with each conversation.

One afternoon, as Sarah was sitting on the porch, her phone rang. It was her best friend, Lucy, who lived out of state. They hadn't seen each other in a while, but they stayed in touch regularly.

"Hey, Lucy!" Sarah answered, her voice filled with excitement.

"Hey, Sarah! I just got your message. I can't believe it! You're going to be a mom!" Lucy's voice was filled with joy.

"I know, it's crazy, right?" Sarah laughed. "I'm so excited and nervous at the same time."

"I can only imagine. I'm so happy for you and Jake. You're going to be amazing parents," Lucy said, her voice sincere.

"Thanks, Lucy. It means a lot to hear that. I wish you were here to celebrate with us."

"Me too. But don't worry, I'll be there as soon as I can. I wouldn't miss it for the world," Lucy promised.

After they hung up, Sarah felt a deep sense of gratitude for the people in her life. She knew that this journey would be filled with challenges, but she also knew that she had a strong support system to help her through it.

As the months went by, Sarah and Jake continued to prepare for the arrival of their baby. They attended prenatal classes, read parenting books, and spent countless hours dreaming about their future. The closer they got to the due date, the more real it all became.

One evening, as they were sitting on the porch, watching the sunset, Sarah turned to Jake. "Can you believe how much our lives have changed in just a few months?"

Jake smiled, wrapping his arm around her. "It's been a whirlwind, but I wouldn't have it any other way. I can't wait to meet our little one."

Sarah rested her head on his shoulder, feeling a deep sense of contentment. "Me neither. I'm so glad we're doing this together."

Jake kissed her forehead. "Always, Sarah. We're a team, and we're going to make this work."

As the sun dipped below the horizon, casting a warm glow over the porch, Sarah felt a sense of peace and happiness that she had never known before. She knew that the journey ahead would be filled with ups and downs, but she also knew that she had Jake by her side, and that made all the difference.

In the end, sharing the news had brought them closer to their loved ones and had strengthened their bond as a couple. They were ready to face whatever challenges came their way, knowing that they had the support and love of their family and friends.

As they looked forward to the future, Sarah felt a sense of excitement and anticipation. She was ready to embrace the journey of parenthood, and she knew that with Jake by her side, they could handle anything that came their way.

Chapter 3: The First Trimester

The first trimester of Sarah's pregnancy was a roller coaster of emotions, physical changes, and adjustments. As the weeks passed, she and Jake navigated the joys and challenges of early pregnancy together, growing closer with each new experience.

Sarah's mornings began with the now-familiar wave of nausea. She had heard about morning sickness, but nothing could have prepared her for the relentless queasiness that often lasted well into the afternoon. She found some relief by nibbling on crackers and sipping ginger tea, but the persistent discomfort was a constant reminder of the tiny life growing inside her.

Jake was a steadfast source of support. He would wake up early to make her tea, rubbing her back as she sipped it slowly. "You're doing great, babe," he would whisper, his words a soothing balm against her worries. His patience and understanding helped Sarah navigate the rough mornings, and his encouragement bolstered her spirits.

Their first visit to the doctor was a significant milestone. Dr. Thompson, a warm and experienced obstetrician, greeted them with a reassuring smile. As Sarah lay on the examination table, Jake held her hand tightly. The room was filled with anticipation as Dr. Thompson applied the cool gel to Sarah's abdomen and began the ultrasound.

The screen flickered to life, revealing a tiny, fluttering heartbeat. Sarah's breath caught in her throat, and she glanced at Jake, who had tears in his eyes. "That's our baby," he whispered, his voice thick with emotion.

Dr. Thompson smiled warmly. "Congratulations, Sarah and Jake. Your baby is doing well."

Hearing their baby's heartbeat for the first time was a transformative experience for Sarah. It made everything feel real, tangible. She was carrying a new life, and the responsibility was both exhilarating and daunting. The sound of the heartbeat stayed with her, a constant reminder of the miracle unfolding within her.

As the weeks went by, Sarah's body continued to change. Her clothes began to feel tighter, and she noticed a small but undeniable bump forming. She and Jake marveled at the physical transformation, often spending evenings with their hands on her belly, feeling for any movement.

Their conversations shifted, too. They talked about baby names, debated the merits of different parenting styles, and imagined what their child might be like. Sarah found comfort in these discussions, feeling more connected to both Jake and the baby with each passing day.

Despite the joy, the first trimester also brought its share of challenges. Sarah experienced mood swings that sometimes took her by surprise. One minute she would be laughing, and the next, she would find herself in tears over something seemingly trivial. Jake's unwavering support helped her navigate these emotional ups and downs. He would hold her, listen to her, and remind her that everything she was feeling was normal.

Work became more challenging as well. The fatigue that accompanied the first trimester was relentless. Sarah found it hard to concentrate during meetings, and by mid-afternoon, she often felt completely drained. She confided in her boss, Lisa, who was understanding and supportive. They arranged for Sarah to work from home a few days a week, which made a significant difference.

One day, as Sarah was working from home, she felt an unusual cramping sensation. Panic set in, and she called Jake, her voice trembling. "I'm scared, Jake. Something doesn't feel right."

Jake immediately left work and rushed home. They went to see Dr. Thompson, who reassured them that cramping could be normal in early pregnancy. An ultrasound confirmed that the baby was fine, and Sarah's fears were somewhat alleviated. However, the experience left her feeling vulnerable and anxious about the uncertainties of pregnancy.

To manage her stress, Sarah began practicing prenatal yoga. She joined a class led by a gentle instructor named Maya, who specialized in yoga for expectant mothers. The classes became a sanctuary for Sarah, a place where she could connect with her body and the life growing within her. She also found a sense of community among the other pregnant women in the class, sharing stories and advice.

One evening, after a particularly relaxing yoga session, Sarah sat on the porch with Jake, the setting sun casting a warm glow over their backyard. She placed his hand on her belly, where she had felt a slight flutter earlier.

"Did you feel that?" she asked, her eyes wide with wonder.

Jake's face lit up with excitement. "I think I did. Our baby is saying hello."

Moments like these made the challenges of the first trimester worthwhile. Despite the nausea, the fatigue, and the emotional highs and lows, there were these magical moments of connection that made it all seem like a grand adventure.

As Sarah entered the final weeks of the first trimester, she noticed a gradual improvement in her symptoms. The nausea began to subside, and her energy levels slowly started to return. She felt a renewed sense of vitality, and the small bump on her belly grew more pronounced.

One Saturday morning, Sarah and Jake decided to start working on the nursery. They had chosen a room that caught the morning light, envisioning it as a bright and welcoming space for their baby. They spent the day painting the walls a soft, calming shade of blue and assembling the crib.

As they worked, they talked about their hopes and dreams for their child. "I can't wait to read them bedtime stories," Sarah said, her voice filled with anticipation. "I want them to have a love of books just like we do."

Jake smiled, handing her a brush. "And I can't wait to teach them how to ride a bike and play catch in the backyard."

The nursery gradually took shape, and with each stroke of paint and piece of furniture assembled, Sarah felt more prepared for the journey ahead. It was a tangible expression of their love and commitment, a space where their baby would grow and thrive.

In the evenings, they continued to attend their prenatal classes, learning about childbirth, breastfeeding, and newborn care. The classes were informative and sometimes overwhelming, but they also provided a sense of reassurance. Sarah and Jake felt more confident knowing that they were taking steps to prepare for their baby's arrival.

One night, as they lay in bed, Sarah turned to Jake. "Do you ever feel scared about all of this?"

Jake looked thoughtful for a moment before answering. "Yeah, sometimes. It's a big change, and there's a lot we don't know. But I also feel excited. We're in this together, and I know we'll figure it out."

Sarah nodded, feeling a wave of affection for Jake. His calm and steady presence was a constant source of comfort. "I'm glad we're doing this together," she said softly.

"Me too," Jake replied, kissing her forehead. "We're going to be a great team."

As the first trimester drew to a close, Sarah felt a sense of accomplishment. She had navigated the initial challenges of pregnancy with grace and resilience, and she knew that the journey was just beginning. There would be more hurdles to overcome, but she felt ready to face them with Jake by her side.

One evening, as they sat on the porch watching the stars, Sarah felt a deep sense of gratitude. She thought about how much their lives had changed in such a short time, and how much more they would change in the months to come.

"Do you ever wonder what our baby will be like?" she asked, leaning into Jake's shoulder.

"All the time," Jake replied. "I imagine them running around the yard, laughing and playing. I can't wait to see who they become."

Sarah smiled, closing her eyes and imagining the future they were creating. "Me neither," she whispered. "It's going to be amazing."

As they sat together under the starlit sky, Sarah felt a profound sense of peace. She knew that there would be challenges ahead, but she also knew that she was surrounded by love and support. With Jake by her side and their baby on the way, she felt ready to embrace whatever the future held.

Chapter 4: Doubts and Fears

As the first trimester faded into memory, Sarah found herself wrestling with an unexpected surge of doubts and fears. The initial excitement of discovering her pregnancy had given way to a profound realization of the immense responsibility that lay ahead. This new chapter in her life, filled with anticipation and joy, was also shadowed by anxieties that seemed to creep up on her during quiet moments.

One afternoon, as Sarah sat in the nursery, she felt a wave of doubt wash over her. The room, now painted and furnished, felt both real and surreal. She ran her hand over the crib's smooth wooden surface, her mind racing with questions. Would she be a good mother? Could she handle the sleepless nights, the endless crying, and the myriad challenges of raising a child? The doubts felt heavy, almost suffocating.

Jake found her there, lost in thought. "Hey, you," he said softly, sitting beside her. "What's on your mind?"

Sarah hesitated, unsure of how to put her feelings into words. "I'm just... I'm scared, Jake. What if

I'm not good enough? What if I mess everything up?"

Jake took her hand, his grip firm and reassuring. "You're going to be an amazing mother, Sarah. We're in this together, remember? We'll figure it out, step by step."

His words were comforting, but the doubts lingered. Sarah knew that Jake believed in her, but she wasn't sure she believed in herself. She had always been a planner, someone who thrived on organization and control. But pregnancy and parenthood were unpredictable, filled with uncertainties that she couldn't plan for.

The next few days were a blur of emotions. Sarah found herself on edge, her moods swinging wildly. One evening, she broke down in tears over a small disagreement with Jake about the color of the nursery curtains. It wasn't about the curtains, she realized; it was about everything else that felt overwhelming and beyond her control.

Jake held her as she cried, his own eyes filled with concern. "We don't have to have all the answers right now, Sarah. We just have to take it one day at a time."

Despite his reassurances, Sarah's fears persisted. She began to doubt her ability to balance work and motherhood, to maintain her relationship with Jake, and to be the kind of mother she wanted to be. These fears gnawed at her, making her question everything.

One night, unable to sleep, Sarah got up and went to the living room. She sat on the couch, her mind racing. She thought about her own childhood, about her mother and the sacrifices she had made. She wondered if she could be as selfless, as nurturing.

Her mother, Linda, had always seemed to have it all together. She had juggled work, family, and countless responsibilities with grace. Sarah picked up the phone and called her, needing to hear her mother's voice.

"Hi, Mom," she said when Linda answered. "I'm sorry it's so late. I just… I needed to talk."

Linda's voice was warm and soothing. "It's okay, honey. What's going on?"

"I'm scared, Mom," Sarah admitted, her voice trembling. "I don't know if I can do this. What if I'm not good enough?"

There was a pause on the other end of the line, and then Linda spoke, her tone gentle but firm. "Sarah, every new mother feels that way. It's completely normal to have doubts and fears. But you have to trust yourself. You're stronger than you think, and you have Jake to support you."

Sarah took a deep breath, feeling a bit of the weight lift off her shoulders. "Thanks, Mom. I just needed to hear that."

Over the next few weeks, Sarah tried to focus on the positives. She threw herself into preparing for the baby, reading books, and attending prenatal classes. She found comfort in the knowledge she gained, each piece of information helping to quell her fears bit by bit.

Jake continued to be her rock, his unwavering support a constant source of strength. They spent evenings talking about their hopes and dreams for the baby, imagining the future with a mix of excitement and trepidation. These conversations helped to ground Sarah, reminding her of the love and partnership they shared.

But even with Jake's support, Sarah couldn't shake the feeling that she was unprepared. She found herself questioning every decision, every plan. One afternoon, while browsing through a baby store, she felt overwhelmed by the sheer number of choices. Should they use cloth diapers or disposable ones? What kind of stroller was best? The questions felt endless, and each decision seemed fraught with the potential for making a mistake.

Feeling the pressure build, Sarah called her friend Emily, who had recently had a baby. They met for coffee, and as they sat in the café, Sarah poured out her fears.

"I just don't know if I'm ready for this, Emily. There's so much to think about, so much to decide. What if I choose the wrong things? What if I'm not a good mother?"

Emily listened patiently, her own experience lending her a sympathetic ear. "Sarah, it's perfectly normal to feel this way. I felt the same before Lucas was born. The truth is, there's no perfect way to do this. You just have to do your best and trust your instincts."

Her words were comforting, a reminder that Sarah wasn't alone in her fears. She wasn't the first woman to feel this way, and she wouldn't be the last. She realized that she needed to be kinder to herself, to allow herself to make mistakes and learn from them.

As the weeks passed, Sarah began to find a rhythm. She focused on the small victories, the moments of joy that reminded her why she was on this journey. The first time she felt the baby move was a revelation, a fluttering sensation that made her laugh with surprise and delight.

"Jake, come here!" she called, grabbing his hand and placing it on her belly. "Do you feel that?"

Jake's eyes widened as he felt the tiny movements. "Wow, that's incredible," he said, his voice filled with wonder. "Our baby is really in there."

Moments like these helped to quiet Sarah's doubts. She began to embrace the journey, accepting that it would be filled with uncertainties and challenges. She found solace in her support system—Jake, her family, her friends—and in the knowledge that she wasn't alone.

One evening, as they sat on the porch watching the sunset, Sarah turned to Jake. "I've been thinking a lot about everything lately. About my fears and doubts."

Jake looked at her, his expression thoughtful. "And what have you concluded?"

Sarah smiled, feeling a sense of peace settle over her. "That it's okay to be scared. It's okay to have doubts. But I know we'll get through this together. We'll figure it out, one step at a time."

Jake squeezed her hand, his eyes filled with love and reassurance. "We will. We're a team, remember?"

Sarah nodded, feeling a renewed sense of confidence. She knew that the journey ahead would be challenging, but she also knew that she had the strength and support to face whatever came her way. As she looked at the horizon, she felt a sense of hope and anticipation for the future they were building together.

The weeks continued to pass, and Sarah found herself growing more comfortable with the idea of motherhood. She still had moments of doubt, but they were tempered by the growing connection she felt with her baby and the unwavering support of Jake and her loved ones.

One morning, as she stood in the nursery, Sarah felt a surge of emotion. She placed her hands on her belly, feeling the life within her. "We're going to be okay," she whispered, her voice filled with determination. "We're going to figure this out together."

In that moment, she knew that she was ready to embrace the journey ahead, with all its challenges and uncertainties. She was ready to face her fears, to trust herself, and to believe in the strength and love that had brought her to this point.

As the second trimester loomed on the horizon, Sarah felt a sense of anticipation. She was ready to take the next steps, to continue preparing for the arrival of their baby. She knew that there would be more doubts and fears along the way, but she also knew that she had the resilience and support to face them head-on.

With Jake by her side and their baby growing stronger every day, Sarah felt a renewed sense of purpose and determination. She was ready to embrace the journey of motherhood, one step at a time, with all its challenges, joys, and uncertainties.

Chapter 5: Planning for the Future

As Sarah entered her second trimester, a renewed sense of energy and optimism washed over her. The lingering nausea had mostly subsided, and her baby bump was growing more prominent. It was time to start planning for the future in earnest, a task that both excited and intimidated her.

The first major project was the nursery. Though they had already painted the walls and set up the basics, there were still plenty of details to finalize. One Saturday morning, Sarah and Jake decided to visit a nearby baby store to pick out the remaining items they needed.

The store was a wonderland of baby gear: rows of cribs, strollers, high chairs, and toys. Sarah felt a mix of excitement and overwhelm as she and Jake navigated the aisles. They carefully selected a soft, cloud-themed mobile for the crib, a rocking chair for late-night feedings, and a set of adorable animal-themed bedding.

"This is really happening," Jake said, his eyes gleaming as he inspected a set of colorful onesies. "Our baby is going to love this stuff."

Sarah smiled, feeling the warmth of his enthusiasm. "It's starting to feel real, isn't it?"

They spent the afternoon arranging their purchases in the nursery. Jake assembled the rocking chair, and Sarah carefully placed the mobile over the crib. As she stepped back to admire their handiwork, she felt a surge of pride and anticipation.

Next on their list was baby-proofing the house. They had heard countless horror stories from friends and family about the dangers lurking in seemingly innocuous places. Sarah and Jake made a checklist of tasks: installing safety gates, securing cabinets, and covering electrical outlets.

One weekend, they tackled the project with determination. Jake installed safety latches on the kitchen cabinets while Sarah padded the sharp corners of their coffee table. They tested every latch and gate, making sure everything was secure. It was tedious work, but the thought of their baby's safety made it worthwhile.

As they worked, they discussed other preparations they needed to make. "We should start thinking about childcare," Sarah said, glancing at Jake. "Do we want to look into daycare, or should we consider a nanny?"

Jake nodded thoughtfully. "Maybe we can visit a few places and see what feels right. It might be good to have a backup plan in case one of us needs to go back to work sooner than expected."

They scheduled visits to several local daycare centers and interviewed a few potential nannies. The process was enlightening and sometimes overwhelming. Each option had its pros and cons, and they took their time weighing each one carefully.

One rainy afternoon, they visited a highly recommended daycare center. The facility was bright and cheerful, filled with the laughter of children. The director gave them a tour, explaining their curriculum and policies. Sarah and Jake were impressed by the center's emphasis on early childhood education and the friendly, attentive staff.

"I think this could be a good fit," Sarah said as they drove home. "It feels safe, and the kids seem happy."

Jake agreed. "Let's keep it on our list. We still have a few more to visit, but this one definitely stands out."

They continued their search, eventually narrowing their options to two excellent choices. It was a relief to have a plan in place, though the decision still weighed heavily on Sarah's mind. The thought of leaving their baby in someone else's care was daunting, but she knew it was a necessary step in balancing their lives and responsibilities.

Amidst the practical preparations, Sarah and Jake also spent time discussing their hopes and dreams for their child. They talked about the values they wanted to instill, the traditions they hoped to uphold, and the kind of parents they aspired to be.

One evening, as they sat by the fire, Sarah broached a topic that had been on her mind for a while. "Jake, have you thought about how we're going to handle work once the baby is here? I've been wondering if I should take an extended leave or maybe even consider working part-time."

Jake looked pensive. "I've been thinking about it too. We're going to have to make some adjustments, but I know we'll find a way to make it work. Maybe we can talk to our employers about flexible schedules or remote work options."

Sarah appreciated Jake's practical approach. They decided to speak with their respective bosses about their plans. Sarah's boss, Lisa, was supportive and agreed to explore options for extended leave and flexible hours. Jake's employer was also accommodating, offering to let him work from home a few days a week once the baby arrived.

These arrangements provided a sense of relief and allowed Sarah and Jake to envision a balanced approach to work and parenting. They knew it wouldn't be easy, but having supportive employers made a world of difference.

As the weeks went by, they also started to think about their finances. Sarah and Jake sat down one evening with a stack of bills and a budget spreadsheet. They reviewed their expenses, considered the costs of raising a child, and made plans to save for the future.

"We should start a college fund," Jake suggested. "It's never too early to start saving."

Sarah agreed. "And we need to update our wills and get life insurance. We have to make sure our baby is taken care of, no matter what happens."

They reached out to a financial advisor, who helped them set up a comprehensive plan. It was another step in preparing for their new reality, and it gave them a sense of security knowing they were taking proactive measures to protect their family's future.

Beyond the practicalities, Sarah and Jake also took time to enjoy the pregnancy journey. They attended prenatal classes, where they learned about childbirth, breastfeeding, and newborn care. These classes not only provided valuable information but also brought them closer together as they practiced breathing techniques and labor positions.

One memorable class focused on bonding with the baby before birth. The instructor encouraged the parents-to-be to talk, sing, and read to their unborn babies. That evening, Sarah and Jake sat on the couch, each holding a children's book. They took turns reading aloud, feeling a bit silly but also deeply connected to their baby.

"Goodnight Moon was one of my favorites growing up," Sarah said, smiling as she read the familiar lines. "I can't wait to share it with our little one."

Jake nodded, his hand resting on Sarah's belly. "Our baby is going to know all the best stories."

These moments of connection helped to alleviate Sarah's lingering doubts and fears. She felt more confident and prepared with each passing day, bolstered by the love and support of Jake and their shared commitment to their growing family.

As they moved through the second trimester, they also made time for themselves as a couple. They went on date nights, enjoyed long walks in the park, and talked about their dreams for the future. These moments of intimacy and connection were a reminder that their relationship was the foundation upon which they were building their family.

One weekend, they decided to take a short getaway to a cozy cabin in the mountains. It was a chance to relax, unwind, and enjoy each other's company before their lives became even busier. They spent their days hiking, cooking together, and talking about their hopes and dreams.

On the last evening of their trip, they sat on the porch, wrapped in blankets as they watched the stars. Sarah felt a deep sense of contentment as she leaned against Jake.

"This is nice," she said softly. "I'm glad we took this time for ourselves."

Jake kissed the top of her head. "Me too. It's important to remember that we're a team, and we need to take care of each other as well as our baby."

Their getaway left them feeling refreshed and more connected than ever. They returned home with a renewed sense of purpose, ready to tackle the remaining preparations for their baby's arrival.

As the weeks continued to pass, Sarah found herself feeling more confident and excited. The baby's movements grew stronger and more frequent, a constant reminder of the life growing inside her. She and Jake spent hours talking to their baby, playing music, and imagining the future.

One evening, as they sat in the nursery, Jake placed his hand on Sarah's belly. "You know, I think our baby is going to be a little musician," he said, smiling. "They always seem to move the most when we play music."

Sarah laughed, feeling a kick beneath Jake's hand. "Maybe we'll have a future rock star on our hands."

Their conversations about the future were filled with joy and anticipation. They imagined first steps, first words, and all the milestones to come. Each day brought them closer to meeting their baby, and they couldn't wait to start this new chapter of their lives.

As they moved toward the end of the second trimester, Sarah and Jake felt a deep sense of readiness. They had planned, prepared, and supported each other through the ups and downs of pregnancy. They knew there would be challenges ahead, but they also knew that they had the strength, love, and resilience to face them together.

With each passing day, their excitement grew. They were ready to welcome their baby into the world, to embrace the joys and challenges of parenthood, and to build a future filled with love, laughter, and countless precious moments.

Chapter 6: The Second Trimester

The second trimester marked a period of growth, change, and anticipation for Sarah and Jake. Sarah's body continued to transform, her baby bump becoming more pronounced each day. The initial symptoms of pregnancy, such as morning sickness and fatigue, had largely subsided, replaced by a sense of renewed energy and optimism.

One morning, as Sarah stood in front of the mirror, she marveled at her reflection. Her belly was round and firm, a tangible reminder of the life growing inside her. She felt a flutter of excitement mixed with a sense of wonder. She was now visibly pregnant, and with each passing day, she felt more connected to her baby.

Jake walked into the bedroom, a cup of tea in hand. "Morning, beautiful," he said, placing the cup on the bedside table. He wrapped his arms around Sarah from behind, resting his hands on her belly. "How are you feeling today?"

Sarah leaned back into him, savoring the warmth of his embrace. "I'm feeling good," she replied, a smile spreading across her face. "It's amazing to see how much I've grown. And I felt the baby move again last night."

Jake's eyes lit up with excitement. "Really? I can't wait to feel it too. Our little one is getting stronger every day."

The baby's movements were a source of endless fascination and joy for both Sarah and Jake. Each kick and flutter brought a sense of connection and anticipation. They spent evenings on the couch, Jake's hand resting on Sarah's belly, hoping to feel the baby's movements together. These moments were intimate and filled with a profound sense of love and wonder.

During the second trimester, Sarah and Jake also attended regular prenatal appointments. These visits to the doctor were both reassuring and informative. They looked forward to hearing their baby's heartbeat and seeing the ultrasound images that provided a glimpse into their baby's world.

One afternoon, they arrived at the clinic for a particularly significant appointment. Sarah was scheduled for an anatomy scan, a detailed ultrasound that would provide a comprehensive look at their baby's development. As they sat in the waiting room, Sarah felt a mix of excitement and nervousness.

Jake squeezed her hand. "Everything's going to be fine," he said, his voice calm and reassuring. "Our baby is strong and healthy."

When they were called into the examination room, the technician greeted them warmly and instructed Sarah to lie down on the table. She applied a cool gel to Sarah's belly and began the scan. The room was filled with the rhythmic sound of the baby's heartbeat, a comforting and steady thump that echoed in Sarah's ears.

As the technician moved the probe across Sarah's belly, the screen displayed images of their baby. Sarah and Jake watched in awe as they saw tiny fingers and toes, a delicate profile, and the fluttering of a little heart. The technician pointed out various features, explaining the baby's growth and development.

"Everything looks great," she said with a smile. "Your baby is developing perfectly."

Sarah felt a wave of relief wash over her. She glanced at Jake, who was beaming with pride. "I can't believe how much we can see," Sarah said, her voice filled with wonder. "It's like meeting our baby for the first time."

Jake nodded, his eyes glued to the screen. "It's incredible. I can't wait to hold our little one in my arms."

The second trimester was also a time for Sarah and Jake to deepen their bond as a couple. They made a conscious effort to spend quality time together, knowing that their lives would become even busier once the baby arrived. They went on date nights, took long walks in the park, and enjoyed quiet evenings at home, talking about their hopes and dreams for the future.

One weekend, they decided to take a short trip to a nearby beach town. It was a chance to relax and unwind, to enjoy each other's company away from the hustle and bustle of daily life. They strolled along the shoreline, hand in hand, the salty breeze ruffling their hair.

As they sat on the sand, watching the waves crash against the shore, Sarah felt a deep sense of peace. "This is nice," she said, leaning her head on Jake's shoulder. "It's good to take a break and just be together."

Jake kissed the top of her head. "I couldn't agree more. These moments are precious, and I'm grateful for every one of them."

Their trip to the beach was a reminder of the importance of savoring the present, of cherishing the journey they were on together. It was a time to reflect on how far they had come and to look forward to the exciting future that awaited them.

Back at home, Sarah and Jake continued to prepare for their baby's arrival. They finalized their childcare plans, set up the nursery, and attended prenatal classes. These classes provided valuable information and helped them feel more confident and prepared.

One evening, as they practiced breathing techniques and labor positions, Sarah couldn't help but laugh. "Can you believe we're doing this?" she said, her eyes sparkling with amusement. "It feels a bit surreal."

Jake grinned. "I know, right? But it's all part of the journey. We're learning and growing together, and that's what matters."

Their classes also introduced them to other expectant parents, creating a sense of community and support. They exchanged tips and stories, finding comfort in knowing they were not alone in their experiences. These connections provided a sense of camaraderie and reassurance, a reminder that they were all in this together.

As the second trimester progressed, Sarah and Jake also made time to connect with their families. They visited Sarah's parents one weekend, bringing them up to date on their preparations and sharing ultrasound photos. Linda and Robert were thrilled to see the images, their excitement palpable.

"I can't wait to meet my grandbaby," Linda said, her eyes misting with tears. "You're going to be wonderful parents."

Sarah felt a lump in her throat. "Thanks, Mom. Your support means the world to us."

They also spent time with Jake's parents, who were equally enthusiastic. "We've been working on a little surprise for the nursery," Jake's mother, Carol, said with a twinkle in her eye. "Can we show you?"

Curious, Sarah and Jake followed Carol and Tom to their car. They opened the trunk to reveal a beautifully hand-carved wooden rocking horse. It was a labor of love, crafted by Tom over several months.

"This is amazing," Sarah said, her voice filled with gratitude. "Thank you so much. Our baby is going to love it."

Tom smiled, his eyes crinkling at the corners. "We wanted to give you something special, something that could be passed down through the generations."

The rocking horse found a place of honor in the nursery, a symbol of the love and support that surrounded Sarah, Jake, and their baby. It was a reminder that they were part of a larger family, one that was eagerly awaiting the arrival of the newest member.

As the weeks turned into months, Sarah continued to experience the physical changes and emotional milestones of pregnancy. She marveled at her growing belly, felt the baby's increasingly strong movements, and reveled in the support and love that enveloped her.

One evening, as she lay in bed, Sarah felt a particularly strong kick. She placed Jake's hand on her belly, and they both felt the baby's movements.

It was a powerful moment, a tangible connection to the life they had created.

"Can you believe we're going to be parents soon?" Sarah whispered, her voice filled with awe.

Jake nodded, his eyes shining with emotion. "It's the most incredible thing. I can't wait to meet our baby and start this new chapter together."

Their conversations often turned to the future, to the dreams and aspirations they held for their child. They talked about the values they wanted to instill, the traditions they hoped to uphold, and the kind of parents they aspired to be.

"We want to give our baby the best start in life," Sarah said one evening as they sat on the porch, watching the sunset. "But we also need to remember to be kind to ourselves. We're going to make mistakes, and that's okay."

Jake squeezed her hand. "Absolutely. We'll learn as we go, and we'll support each other every step of the way."

As the second trimester drew to a close, Sarah and Jake felt a deep sense of readiness. They had prepared, planned, and connected with each other and their support system. They knew there would be challenges ahead, but they also knew they had the strength, love, and resilience to face them together.

With each passing day, their excitement grew. They were ready to welcome their baby into the world, to embrace the joys and challenges of parenthood, and to build a future filled with love, laughter, and countless precious moments.

The second trimester had been a time of growth, preparation, and deepening bonds. It had brought them closer together as a couple and as a family, and it had strengthened their resolve to face the future with hope and determination.

As they looked ahead to the final trimester, Sarah and Jake felt a sense of anticipation and excitement. They were ready to continue this journey, to embrace the unknown, and to welcome their baby into their lives with open hearts and boundless love.

Chapter 7: Changes in Relationships

As Sarah's pregnancy progressed, she found that her relationships with those around her were undergoing significant changes. This chapter in her life was not just about her transformation into motherhood but also about how her connections with her partner, family, friends, and even herself evolved.

Sarah's bond with Jake continued to deepen. They had always been close, but the shared experience of preparing for their baby's arrival brought them even closer. They found themselves spending more time together, whether it was working on the nursery, attending prenatal classes, or simply enjoying quiet evenings at home.

One evening, as they sat on the porch sipping hot cocoa, Sarah turned to Jake. "You know, I feel like we're becoming a stronger team," she said, her voice filled with warmth. "I'm grateful for you every day."

Jake smiled and took her hand. "I feel the same way. This journey has been incredible, and I can't imagine doing it with anyone else."

Their conversations often revolved around their hopes and dreams for their family. They discussed parenting philosophies, shared childhood memories, and imagined what their baby might be like. These discussions brought a sense of unity and shared purpose, reinforcing their commitment to each other and their growing family.

However, it wasn't all smooth sailing. Pregnancy brought its own set of challenges, and sometimes, the stress of impending parenthood would lead to disagreements. One afternoon, as they were organizing the nursery, they found themselves at odds over where to place the crib.

"I think it should go by the window," Jake suggested. "It'll get plenty of natural light there."

Sarah shook her head. "But I read that it's better to keep the crib away from windows to avoid drafts. Plus, what if there's a risk of the baby pulling on the blinds when they get older?"

Jake frowned. "I hadn't thought of that. But the room is so small; it's hard to find a perfect spot."

They stood there, staring at the crib and trying to find a solution. After a moment of silence, Sarah took a deep breath. "Let's take a break and think it over. We can come back to it later."

Jake nodded, his expression softening. "Good idea. We'll figure it out together."

This willingness to communicate and compromise became a cornerstone of their relationship. They learned to navigate disagreements with patience and understanding, recognizing that their love and commitment were stronger than any temporary conflict.

Sarah's relationships with her family also evolved during her pregnancy. Her parents, Linda and Robert, were a constant source of support and encouragement. They were thrilled about becoming grandparents and often shared advice and stories from when Sarah was a baby.

One weekend, Sarah and Jake visited Linda and Robert's house for a family dinner. As they sat around the table, enjoying a home-cooked meal, Linda shared a story about Sarah's first steps.

"You were so determined," Linda said, her eyes twinkling with nostalgia. "You would pull yourself up on the furniture and wobble around, never giving up. I see that same determination in you now."

Sarah smiled, touched by her mother's words. "Thanks, Mom. Your stories always make me feel more confident about this whole parenting thing."

Robert chimed in, his voice filled with pride. "You're going to be amazing parents. And remember, we're always here if you need help or advice."

Their support gave Sarah a sense of security, knowing that she wasn't alone in this journey. She felt a renewed appreciation for her parents and the values they had instilled in her, values she hoped to pass on to her own child.

Jake's parents, Carol and Tom, were equally enthusiastic about their grandchild. They visited often, bringing gifts and offering their assistance with preparations. One afternoon, they arrived with a beautifully hand-knitted blanket that Carol had made.

"I hope the baby likes it," Carol said, her eyes shining with love. "I put a lot of heart into this."

Sarah ran her fingers over the soft yarn, feeling the warmth and care woven into every stitch. "It's perfect, Carol. Thank you so much."

Tom added, "We're here for you both, every step of the way. If you need anything, don't hesitate to call."

These visits strengthened Sarah's bond with Jake's parents and made her feel even more connected to their family. She appreciated their kindness and generosity, knowing that their support would be invaluable in the months and years ahead.

Sarah's friendships also experienced a shift during her pregnancy. Some friends were incredibly supportive, excitedly sharing in her joy and offering help and advice. Others seemed to pull away, unsure of how to relate to her new reality.

Her best friend, Emily, was a constant source of support. They had been friends since college, and their bond had only grown stronger over the years. Emily was thrilled about Sarah's pregnancy and often checked in to see how she was doing.

One afternoon, they met for coffee at their favorite café. As they sipped their drinks, Emily leaned in, her eyes sparkling with excitement. "How's my favorite mama-to-be doing?"

Sarah smiled, grateful for Emily's enthusiasm. "I'm doing well, thanks. It's been a whirlwind, but I'm starting to feel more prepared."

Emily reached across the table and squeezed Sarah's hand. "You're going to be an amazing mom. And I'm here for you, every step of the way."

Their conversations ranged from baby names to nursery themes, to more personal reflections on how Sarah was feeling. Emily's support was a lifeline, providing Sarah with a sense of continuity and reassurance.

However, not all friendships were as easy to navigate. Some friends seemed distant, unsure of how to connect with Sarah's new reality. She noticed that invitations to social events became less frequent, and some friends seemed uncomfortable discussing her pregnancy.

One evening, Sarah confided in Jake about her feelings of isolation. "I feel like some of my friends don't know how to relate to me anymore. It's like I'm living in a different world."

Jake wrapped his arms around her, offering comfort. "It's a big change, not just for us but for everyone around us. Give it time. True friends will find a way to stay connected."

Sarah took his words to heart, reaching out to her friends and finding new ways to connect. She organized casual get-togethers, inviting friends over for movie nights and game evenings. These gatherings helped bridge the gap, reminding her friends that while her life was changing, her core self remained the same.

In addition to her relationships with others, Sarah also noticed changes in her relationship with herself. Pregnancy had brought about a profound transformation, both physically and emotionally. She found herself reflecting on her identity, her values, and the kind of mother she wanted to be.

One evening, as she sat in the nursery, Sarah took a moment to journal her thoughts. She wrote about her hopes and fears, her dreams for her child, and the lessons she had learned so far.

"I want to be a mother who is patient and kind," she wrote. "Someone who listens, who supports, who loves unconditionally. I want to teach my child the importance of empathy, resilience, and courage."

Writing these thoughts down helped Sarah clarify her vision for the future. It also provided a sense of peace, reminding her that she was capable of navigating this journey with grace and strength.

As the second trimester progressed, Sarah continued to grow and evolve. She found a balance between preparing for the future and savoring the present. She embraced the changes in her relationships, recognizing that they were an integral part of her journey into motherhood.

One weekend, she and Jake attended a prenatal yoga class together. The class focused on relaxation and connection, helping expectant parents bond with their babies and each other. As they moved through the gentle poses, Sarah felt a deep sense of peace and unity.

After the class, they sat in the park, enjoying the warm afternoon sun. "That was wonderful," Sarah said, leaning against Jake. "I feel so much more connected to you and our baby."

Jake smiled, his eyes filled with love. "Me too. This journey has been incredible, and I'm grateful for every moment."

Their bond had strengthened through the shared experience of pregnancy, and they felt ready to face the challenges and joys of parenthood together. They knew that their relationships with each other and those around them would continue to evolve, but they were confident in their ability to navigate these changes with love and resilience.

As Sarah looked ahead to the final trimester, she felt a deep sense of anticipation and excitement. She was ready to embrace the next chapter, to welcome her baby into the world, and to continue growing and evolving as a mother, partner, and friend.

With each passing day, her relationships continued to deepen and transform, reflecting the profound journey she was on. And through it all, she felt a sense of gratitude for the love and support that surrounded her, knowing that she was never alone on this incredible journey of growth and change.

Chapter 8: The Gender Reveal

The anticipation of discovering their baby's gender was a thrilling part of Sarah and Jake's pregnancy journey. From the moment they found out they were expecting, the question of whether they would have a boy or a girl lingered in their minds, adding an extra layer of excitement to the process.

As the date for their gender reveal appointment approached, Sarah and Jake decided they wanted to share this special moment with their family and close friends. They planned a small gathering at their home, envisioning a celebration filled with joy, love, and anticipation.

The week leading up to the event was a whirlwind of preparations. Sarah and Jake worked together to organize the party, carefully selecting decorations, planning games, and deciding on a menu. They wanted everything to be perfect, creating an atmosphere that reflected their happiness and excitement.

Sarah's mother, Linda, offered to help with the preparations. She arrived at their house one morning, her arms filled with supplies. "I brought some decorations and a few ideas for games," she said, her eyes sparkling with enthusiasm.

Sarah welcomed her mother's help, grateful for her support. "Thanks, Mom. I'm so glad you're here. This is going to be such a special day."

Together, they transformed the living room and backyard into a festive space, adorned with blue and pink decorations. Streamers, balloons, and banners added a cheerful touch, and a large "Boy or Girl?" sign took center stage.

As they worked, Linda shared stories from her own experiences with gender reveals and baby showers. "We didn't have big parties like this when I was pregnant with you," she said with a smile. "But I remember feeling the same excitement and anticipation. It's such a magical time."

Sarah nodded, feeling a deep connection to her mother. "I'm so happy you're here to share this with us. It means a lot."

Jake's parents, Carol and Tom, also arrived early to help with the preparations. Carol brought a beautifully decorated cake, its frosting concealing the secret that would soon be revealed. "I can't wait to see everyone's reactions," she said, placing the cake on the table. "This is going to be so much fun."

Tom set up a makeshift photo booth in the backyard, complete with props and a backdrop. "We'll capture all the special moments," he said, adjusting his camera. "These are memories you'll cherish forever."

As the day of the gender reveal party arrived, Sarah and Jake felt a mix of excitement and nervousness. They had decided to keep the baby's gender a surprise even from themselves, trusting their doctor to deliver the results to Carol, who would prepare the cake.

Guests began to arrive, filling the house with laughter and chatter. Sarah's best friend, Emily, was among the first to arrive, carrying a gift bag. "I brought something for the baby, whether it's a boy or a girl," she said, hugging Sarah. "I'm so excited for you!"

Sarah and Jake mingled with their guests, feeling the love and support of their family and friends. The atmosphere was filled with anticipation, everyone eager to find out whether they were expecting a little boy or girl.

As the party got underway, Linda led the guests in a series of fun games. They played "Guess the Gender," where everyone wrote down their predictions and placed them in a jar. They also had a diaper-changing race, where guests competed to see who could diaper a baby doll the fastest.

Laughter filled the air as everyone joined in the fun. The games were a lighthearted way to celebrate the impending arrival of Sarah and Jake's baby, and they provided an opportunity for everyone to bond and share in the excitement.

Finally, it was time for the big reveal. Carol brought out the cake, its pristine frosting hiding the secret within. She placed it on the table, and everyone gathered around, their faces alight with anticipation.

Sarah and Jake stood side by side, holding a knife. "Are you ready?" Jake whispered, his voice tinged with excitement.

Sarah nodded, her heart pounding. "Let's do this."

Together, they cut into the cake, revealing a burst of color inside. The room erupted in cheers and applause as the answer was unveiled: pink frosting filled the center of the cake, indicating they were having a baby girl.

Tears of joy filled Sarah's eyes as she turned to Jake. "We're having a girl!" she exclaimed, her voice filled with wonder and happiness.

Jake's eyes were misty as he hugged her tightly. "I can't believe it. We're going to have a daughter."

Their friends and family surrounded them, offering hugs and congratulations. Emily handed Sarah a small, pink onesie she had brought as a gift. "I had a feeling it was a girl," she said with a grin. "She's going to be so loved."

The rest of the party was a blur of joy and celebration. Guests took turns at the photo booth, posing with "Team Pink" and "Team Blue" signs. Linda and Carol shared stories and advice, their excitement for their future granddaughter evident in their every word.

As the sun set and the party wound down, Sarah and Jake found a quiet moment together. They sat on the porch, watching the sky turn shades of orange and pink. Sarah leaned her head on Jake's shoulder, feeling a deep sense of contentment.

"This has been an amazing day," she said softly. "I feel so blessed to have such wonderful family and friends."

Jake kissed the top of her head. "Me too. And now we know we're having a little girl. Our family is growing, and it's the best feeling in the world."

They sat in comfortable silence, their hearts full of love and anticipation. The gender reveal had been a beautiful milestone in their journey, a moment of pure joy that they would remember forever.

In the days that followed, Sarah and Jake continued to prepare for their baby girl's arrival. They painted the nursery a soft, soothing shade of pink and filled it with delicate, floral decorations. They shopped for tiny dresses and blankets, imagining their daughter in each outfit.

Sarah found herself daydreaming about the future, picturing the special moments they would share with their daughter. She thought about teaching her to read, taking her on walks in the park, and watching her grow and discover the world.

Jake was equally excited, often talking about the adventures they would have as a family. "I can't wait to take her camping," he said one evening as they sat in the nursery. "We'll teach her to love nature and explore the world."

Sarah smiled, her heart swelling with love for Jake and their unborn daughter. "She's going to be so lucky to have you as her dad."

As they navigated the final months of pregnancy, Sarah and Jake found themselves even more connected, their shared anticipation bringing them closer together. They continued to attend prenatal classes, learning as much as they could to prepare for their daughter's arrival.

One afternoon, they sat in their living room, sorting through baby clothes and supplies. Sarah held up a tiny pair of pink socks, marveling at their size. "It's hard to believe she's going to be this small," she said, her voice filled with wonder.

Jake smiled, taking the socks from her. "And she's going to grow so fast. We'll cherish every moment."

Their evenings were often spent in the nursery, reading books and imagining the future. Sarah found comfort in these quiet moments, feeling a deep sense of peace and readiness.

As they approached the end of the second trimester, they scheduled another ultrasound to check on their baby's development. The appointment was a chance to see their daughter again and ensure that everything was progressing smoothly.

The ultrasound technician greeted them warmly as they entered the examination room. "Ready to see your little girl again?" she asked, preparing the equipment.

Sarah lay back on the table, feeling a flutter of excitement. The technician applied the gel to her belly and began the scan. The room filled with the rhythmic sound of the baby's heartbeat, a comforting and familiar thump.

As the images appeared on the screen, Sarah and Jake watched in awe. Their daughter's tiny form was clearly visible, her movements graceful and active. The technician pointed out various features, explaining the baby's growth and development.

"Everything looks great," she said with a smile. "Your little girl is healthy and growing beautifully."

Sarah felt a wave of relief and happiness. She glanced at Jake, who was beaming with pride. "She's perfect," Sarah whispered, her heart full.

Jake nodded, his eyes never leaving the screen. "Absolutely perfect."

The ultrasound was another cherished moment, a reminder of the miracle growing inside Sarah. As they left the clinic, hand in hand, they felt more ready than ever to welcome their daughter into the world.

The gender reveal had been a beautiful and memorable event, marking a significant milestone in their journey. It had brought their family and friends together, strengthening their bonds and creating a sense of community and support.

As Sarah and Jake continued to prepare for the arrival of their baby girl, they felt a deep sense of gratitude and anticipation. They knew that the road ahead would be filled with challenges and joys, and they were ready to face it together, hand in hand, with love and determination.

Chapter 9: Unexpected Complications

As Sarah entered the third trimester of her pregnancy, she felt a mix of excitement and nervousness. The due date was approaching, and she and Jake were busy with final preparations. The nursery was ready, their hospital bag packed, and they had attended all the prenatal classes. They felt prepared for the arrival of their daughter, but life had a way of throwing curveballs.

One morning, Sarah woke up feeling unusually fatigued. She had been experiencing some swelling in her feet and hands, but she attributed it to the typical discomforts of late pregnancy. However, today felt different. Her head was pounding, and she noticed her vision was slightly blurry. Concerned, she decided to call her obstetrician.

Dr. Patel, her obstetrician, advised her to come in for a check-up. Jake took the day off work to accompany her, sensing her anxiety. They arrived at the clinic and were promptly taken to an examination room.

Dr. Patel greeted them warmly. "How are you feeling, Sarah?"

Sarah described her symptoms, trying to stay calm. "I've been feeling really tired, and my vision is a bit blurry. I also have some swelling in my feet and hands."

Dr. Patel listened attentively and then took Sarah's blood pressure. Her brow furrowed slightly. "Your blood pressure is quite high, Sarah. I'm going to run a few tests to be sure, but it sounds like you might have preeclampsia."

Sarah's heart sank. She had read about preeclampsia and knew it could be serious. "Is the baby going to be okay?" she asked, her voice trembling.

Dr. Patel placed a reassuring hand on Sarah's shoulder. "We're going to monitor you both very closely. If it is preeclampsia, we'll take the necessary steps to ensure the best outcome for you and the baby."

The next few hours were a whirlwind of tests and monitoring. Sarah's blood pressure remained high, and the lab results confirmed Dr. Patel's suspicion. She had preeclampsia, a condition characterized by high blood pressure and signs of damage to another organ system, often the liver or kidneys.

Dr. Patel explained the situation to Sarah and Jake. "Preeclampsia can be dangerous for both mother and baby. We need to monitor you closely and may need to deliver the baby early if your condition worsens."

The news was overwhelming. Sarah felt a mixture of fear and disappointment. She had envisioned a smooth pregnancy and delivery, but now she was facing a serious complication. Jake held her hand, offering silent support as they absorbed the information.

Dr. Patel admitted Sarah to the hospital for closer monitoring. She was placed on bed rest, and her blood pressure was checked regularly. Sarah felt a wave of emotions—fear for her baby's health, anxiety about the potential for an early delivery, and frustration at the sudden change in her pregnancy journey.

The hospital room became their new reality. Nurses came in and out, checking on Sarah and the baby. Jake stayed by her side, offering comfort and reassurance. Despite the uncertainty, their bond grew stronger as they faced this challenge together.

One evening, as they sat in the dimly lit room, Jake tried to lighten the mood. "Remember that camping trip we took last year? The one where it rained the entire time?"

Sarah managed a small smile. "How could I forget? We ended up soaked and miserable, but we laughed the whole time."

Jake chuckled. "We got through that together, and we'll get through this too. We're a team, and we'll face whatever comes our way."

Sarah squeezed his hand, grateful for his unwavering support. "You're right. We'll get through this."

As the days passed, Sarah's condition remained stable but precarious. Dr. Patel visited regularly, keeping them informed about the situation. "We're going to keep monitoring you closely," she said. "If there are any signs of worsening, we'll need to consider delivering the baby early. But for now, rest and try to stay calm."

The waiting was agonizing. Sarah felt helpless, confined to her hospital bed while the world outside continued. She missed the simple pleasures of daily life—walking in the park, cooking dinner with Jake, and even just lounging on the couch.

Her friends and family visited often, bringing flowers, cards, and words of encouragement. Emily came by with a basket of Sarah's favorite snacks. "I know hospital food isn't great, so I brought you some treats," she said with a wink.

Sarah appreciated the gesture. "Thank you, Emily. It means a lot to have you here."

Emily sat by her bedside, chatting and catching up on the latest news. Their conversations provided a welcome distraction from the constant monitoring and medical updates.

Linda and Robert were frequent visitors as well. They brought books and magazines to keep Sarah entertained and shared stories from their own experiences as parents. "You were a handful when you were born," Linda said with a smile. "But we got through it, and so will you."

Sarah drew strength from their stories and their unwavering belief in her ability to handle this challenge. She knew she had a strong support system, and that gave her hope.

Despite the support, there were moments of intense fear and uncertainty. One night, Sarah woke up feeling a sharp pain in her abdomen. She pressed the call button, and within moments, a nurse was at her side.

"What's wrong, Sarah?" the nurse asked, her voice calm and reassuring.

"I have a sharp pain in my abdomen," Sarah replied, trying to stay composed.

The nurse quickly checked her vitals and paged Dr. Patel. Within minutes, Dr. Patel arrived, her expression focused and determined. She examined Sarah and ordered an immediate ultrasound.

The ultrasound technician arrived and performed the scan. As Sarah watched the screen, she saw her baby's tiny form, moving and wriggling. The technician assured her that the baby was okay, but the pain was concerning.

Dr. Patel explained the situation. "The pain could be a sign that your preeclampsia is worsening. We need to monitor you very closely tonight."

The hours that followed were tense. Sarah was given medication to manage the pain, and her blood pressure was monitored continuously. Jake stayed by her side, holding her hand and whispering words of comfort.

As dawn broke, the pain subsided, and Sarah's condition stabilized. Dr. Patel returned with a sense of relief. "The pain seems to have passed, but we need to stay vigilant. You're doing great, Sarah. Just hang in there."

Sarah felt a wave of gratitude for the medical team's care and Jake's unwavering support. She knew she was in good hands, but the uncertainty was draining.

The days turned into weeks, and Sarah remained in the hospital, her condition closely monitored. Despite the challenges, she found moments of joy and hope. She and Jake continued to bond over the experience, their love and commitment growing stronger.

One afternoon, as Sarah lay in bed, Jake surprised her with a small gift. He handed her a beautifully wrapped box. "I know it's not much, but I thought you could use a little pick-me-up."

Sarah opened the box to find a delicate necklace with a pendant shaped like a tiny footprint. She felt tears welling up in her eyes. "It's beautiful, Jake. Thank you."

Jake smiled, his eyes full of love. "I thought it could be a reminder of our little one and the journey we're on. We're going to get through this, and soon we'll be holding our baby girl."

Sarah clutched the necklace, feeling a renewed sense of hope. "I can't wait to meet her. She's going to be so loved."

As the end of the third trimester approached, Dr. Patel made a difficult decision. "Sarah, we need to deliver the baby early. Your condition is stable, but we can't take any risks. We're going to schedule a C-section for tomorrow."

The news was both a relief and a source of anxiety. Sarah knew it was the best decision for her and the baby's health, but the thought of an early delivery was daunting.

Jake held her close, his voice steady and reassuring. "We're going to meet our daughter tomorrow. Everything will be okay."

Sarah took a deep breath, finding strength in his words. "Yes, we're going to meet her. And she's going to be perfect."

The night before the C-section, Sarah and Jake spent a quiet evening together, reflecting on their journey. They talked about their hopes and dreams for their daughter, imagining the life they would build as a family.

The next morning, Sarah was prepped for surgery. The medical team was calm and efficient, explaining each step of the process. Jake was by her side, dressed in scrubs and holding her hand.

As they entered the operating room, Sarah felt a mix of fear and excitement. The lights were bright, and the room buzzed with activity. Dr. Patel greeted her with a reassuring smile. "You're in good hands, Sarah. We're going to take great care of you and your baby."

The procedure began, and Sarah focused on Jake's steady presence beside her. Within minutes, she heard the first cries of their baby girl. Tears streamed down her face as she realized the moment had finally arrived.

Dr. Patel held up their daughter, her tiny form wriggling and crying. "Congratulations, Sarah and Jake. You have a beautiful baby girl."

Jake's eyes filled with tears as he looked at their daughter. "She's perfect," he whispered, his voice choked with emotion.

The medical team quickly assessed the baby's health and then placed her in Sarah's arms. Sarah gazed down at her daughter, feeling a surge of love and protectiveness. "Hello, little one," she whispered. "We've been waiting for you."

The journey had been filled with unexpected complications and challenges, but in that moment, everything felt worth it. Sarah and Jake had navigated the ups and downs together, and now they were holding the precious result of their love and perseverance.

As they looked at their daughter, they knew that their journey was just beginning. There would be more challenges ahead, but they were ready to face them together, as a family. The road had been difficult, but it had led them to this beautiful moment, and they were grateful for every step of the way.

Chapter 10: The Third Trimester

The third trimester marked the home stretch of Sarah's pregnancy, a period filled with anticipation and growing excitement, despite the unexpected complications she faced. With the early delivery of their baby girl, Emma, Sarah and Jake's world was irrevocably changed. The weeks following her birth were a mixture of challenges, triumphs, and an overwhelming sense of love and responsibility.

Back at home, the nursery that had been meticulously prepared for Emma now felt complete with her presence. Sarah and Jake spent countless hours in the cozy, pink room, marveling at their daughter and adjusting to the rhythms of newborn life. Emma's cries, coos, and tiny movements filled their days and nights, a constant reminder of the miracle they had brought into the world.

The first few days were a blur of feedings, diaper changes, and sleepless nights. Sarah's recovery from the C-section added an extra layer of difficulty, but Jake was a steadfast partner, ensuring she had everything she needed while also tending to Emma's needs. The bond between them grew stronger as they navigated the challenges of early parenthood together.

One morning, as sunlight streamed through the nursery window, Jake entered the room to find Sarah cradling Emma in the rocking chair. He smiled, watching the serene scene before him. "How are my girls doing?" he asked softly.

Sarah looked up, exhaustion etched on her face but a smile playing on her lips. "We're doing okay. She just finished eating and finally fell asleep."

Jake knelt beside them, gently stroking Emma's tiny hand. "She's so perfect, Sarah. I can't believe she's here."

"I know," Sarah whispered, her eyes filled with wonder. "Every time I look at her, I feel like my heart might burst."

Despite the challenges, there were moments of pure joy and awe. Sarah and Jake cherished the simple, everyday moments—Emma's first smile, the way she gripped their fingers with surprising strength, the soft sounds she made as she slept. These moments were a balm to the exhaustion and the occasional overwhelm they felt.

Their families were a constant source of support. Linda and Robert visited frequently, bringing homemade meals and offering to watch Emma so Sarah and Jake could get some much-needed rest. Sarah's mother, Linda, was especially attentive, sharing advice and stories from her own experiences as a new mother.

One afternoon, Linda arrived with a batch of freshly baked cookies. "I thought you could use a little treat," she said, placing the cookies on the kitchen counter.

Sarah hugged her mother, grateful for the gesture. "Thanks, Mom. You have no idea how much we appreciate your help."

Linda smiled warmly. "It's my pleasure, sweetheart. I remember how overwhelming those first few weeks can be. Just remember to take care of yourself, too."

Sarah nodded, knowing her mother was right. Self-care often took a backseat in the whirlwind of newborn care, but she was determined to find a balance.

Jake's parents, Carol and Tom, were also regular visitors. Carol, a retired nurse, offered invaluable advice on baby care and helped ease Sarah's concerns about Emma's health and development. "She's doing great," Carol reassured them during one visit. "You're doing everything right."

Tom, meanwhile, enjoyed spending time with his granddaughter, holding her gently and singing lullabies. "You've got a natural touch," Jake remarked one evening as Tom rocked Emma to sleep.

Tom chuckled. "Years of practice, son. She's a little angel."

As the days turned into weeks, Sarah and Jake began to find a rhythm. They learned to communicate more effectively, supporting each other through the highs and lows of parenthood. They discovered the importance of teamwork, dividing responsibilities and ensuring they both had moments to rest and recharge.

One night, as they sat together on the couch, watching Emma sleep in her bassinet, Jake turned to Sarah. "I know this has been tough, but I wouldn't trade it for anything," he said softly. "Seeing you with Emma, being a family—it's everything I ever wanted."

Sarah leaned her head on his shoulder, feeling a deep sense of contentment. "Me too, Jake. She's our little miracle."

As they settled into their new roles, Sarah's focus gradually shifted from immediate recovery to long-term planning. She and Jake began to discuss their future, considering everything from childcare options to career adjustments. Sarah, who had always been driven in her career, found herself reevaluating her priorities in light of motherhood.

One afternoon, while Emma napped, Sarah and Jake sat at the kitchen table, discussing their plans.

"I've been thinking about going back to work part-time," Sarah said, stirring her tea. "I love my job, but I don't want to miss out on these early years with Emma."

Jake nodded thoughtfully. "We can make it work. Maybe I can adjust my schedule, too, so we can share the load."

Their discussions were pragmatic yet filled with hope. They knew balancing careers and parenthood would be challenging, but they were committed to finding a solution that worked for their family.

As Emma grew, Sarah and Jake began to venture out more, introducing her to the world beyond their home. They took her on walks in the park, delighting in her wide-eyed curiosity. They visited friends and family, sharing the joy of their new addition and receiving endless compliments on Emma's adorableness.

One sunny Saturday, they decided to visit the local farmer's market. It was their first major outing as a family, and they were both excited and nervous. Sarah dressed Emma in a cute little outfit, complete with a sunhat to protect her delicate skin.

As they strolled through the market, pushing Emma in her stroller, they felt a sense of normalcy returning. They stopped at various stalls, picking up fresh produce and chatting with vendors. Many people stopped to admire Emma, their faces lighting up at the sight of the tiny baby.

"She's beautiful," an elderly woman said, peering into the stroller. "How old is she?"

"Just a few weeks," Sarah replied, smiling proudly.

The woman's eyes softened. "Enjoy every moment. They grow up so fast."

The outing was a success, and Sarah and Jake returned home feeling more confident and connected. They realized that while their lives had changed dramatically, they could still enjoy the activities they loved, now with Emma by their side.

As the third trimester came to a close, Sarah reflected on the journey they had been through. The unexpected complications had tested their resilience and strength, but they had emerged stronger and more united. The love they felt for Emma was boundless, and it fueled their determination to be the best parents they could be.

One evening, as they prepared for bed, Sarah and Jake stood by Emma's crib, watching her sleep.

The soft glow of the nightlight bathed the room in a warm, gentle light.

"She's our little miracle," Jake whispered, his arm around Sarah's shoulders.

Sarah nodded, feeling tears of joy welling up. "She's everything we ever dreamed of and more."

Their journey was far from over. There would be more challenges, more sleepless nights, and more moments of doubt. But there would also be countless moments of joy, love, and growth. As they looked at their daughter, they knew they were ready for whatever the future held, as long as they faced it together.

In the weeks that followed, Sarah and Jake continued to adapt to their new roles as parents. They cherished the small victories, celebrated milestones, and leaned on each other for support. Their love for Emma deepened with each passing day, and they felt a profound sense of gratitude for the family they had created.

As they navigated the ups and downs of parenthood, they held on to the lessons they had learned during Sarah's pregnancy and the early days of Emma's life. They knew that, no matter what challenges lay ahead, they had the strength, resilience, and love to overcome them.

The third trimester had been a period of growth and transformation, not just for Sarah and Emma, but for their entire family. It had tested their limits and shown them the depths of their love and commitment. And as they looked to the future, they felt ready to embrace it with open hearts, knowing that the journey of parenthood was just beginning.

Chapter 11: Building a Support Network

With Emma's arrival, Sarah and Jake realized the importance of having a strong support network. Navigating the challenges of parenthood, especially with the unexpected complications they had faced, underscored the need for a solid foundation of family, friends, and community. Over the weeks that followed, they took deliberate steps to build and strengthen their support network, ensuring they had the help and resources needed to thrive as a new family.

In the early days after bringing Emma home, Sarah and Jake leaned heavily on their immediate family. Sarah's mother, Linda, was a constant presence, offering not only practical help but also emotional support. She often spent afternoons at their house, rocking Emma to sleep, preparing meals, and sharing invaluable parenting wisdom.

One morning, as Linda prepared breakfast in the kitchen, she glanced over at Sarah, who was nursing Emma on the couch. "You know, you and Jake are doing an amazing job," Linda said, her voice filled with pride.

Sarah smiled, feeling reassured by her mother's words. "Thanks, Mom. I don't know what we would do without you."

Linda walked over, placing a gentle hand on Sarah's shoulder. "That's what family is for. We're here to help you through this."

Jake's parents, Carol and Tom, were also frequent visitors. Carol's experience as a nurse provided an extra layer of confidence for Sarah and Jake. She offered advice on everything from breastfeeding techniques to recognizing the signs of a healthy baby. Tom, meanwhile, enjoyed bonding with his granddaughter, often taking her for walks around the neighborhood in her stroller.

One afternoon, Carol and Tom arrived with a stack of books and a basket of home-cooked meals. "We thought you could use some new reading material and a break from cooking," Carol said, handing the basket to Jake.

Jake grinned, accepting the basket. "You two are lifesavers. Thank you so much."

As the days turned into weeks, Sarah and Jake began to expand their support network beyond immediate family. They reached out to friends, many of whom had young children of their own and could relate to the challenges they were facing.

Emily, Sarah's best friend, was a constant source of encouragement. She visited regularly, bringing laughter and a sense of normalcy to the chaotic early days of parenthood. One evening, she showed up with a bottle of wine and a board game. "I thought you might need a break," Emily said with a wink.

Sarah laughed, feeling a wave of gratitude for her friend. "You're a mind reader, Emily. We could definitely use some fun."

As they sat around the table, chatting and playing the game, Sarah felt a sense of relief. It was a reminder that, despite the demands of parenthood, it was important to take time for themselves and nurture their friendships.

Jake's friends were equally supportive. His best friend, Mark, who had recently become a father himself, offered practical advice and a listening ear. They often met up for coffee or a quick lunch, sharing stories and tips on surviving the early days of fatherhood.

One afternoon, as they sat in a café, Mark leaned in, his voice serious. "Remember, Jake, it's okay to ask for help. We all need it, and there's no shame in admitting you're overwhelmed."

Jake nodded, appreciating Mark's honesty. "Thanks, Mark. It's good to know we're not alone in this."

In addition to family and friends, Sarah and Jake sought out local parenting groups and community resources. They attended a new parents' support group at the local community center, where they met other couples going through similar experiences. The group provided a safe space to share their struggles and triumphs, and they quickly formed connections with other parents.

During one meeting, a fellow new mother named Rachel shared her story of postpartum depression and the importance of seeking help. "It's crucial to take care of your mental health," Rachel said, her voice steady but emotional. "Don't hesitate to reach out if you're struggling."

Sarah felt a deep sense of empathy and understanding. She had experienced moments of anxiety and doubt herself, and hearing Rachel's story reminded her of the importance of self-care and seeking support.

The community center also offered workshops on various parenting topics, from infant CPR to early childhood development. Sarah and Jake attended several of these workshops, eager to learn and feel more confident in their roles as parents.

At one workshop on infant sleep patterns, the instructor emphasized the importance of establishing a routine. "Consistency is key," she explained. "Create a bedtime routine that works for your family and stick to it."

Sarah and Jake took this advice to heart, developing a nightly routine that included a warm bath, a bedtime story, and soothing lullabies. Over time, they noticed a positive change in Emma's sleep patterns, which in turn helped them feel more rested and capable.

As they continued to build their support network, Sarah and Jake also made a conscious effort to maintain open lines of communication with each other. They had always been a strong team, but the demands of parenthood required even more coordination and understanding.

One evening, after Emma had finally fallen asleep, they sat on the couch, reflecting on their journey so far. "I know it's been tough," Jake said, his voice filled with sincerity. "But I'm so grateful to have you by my side."

Sarah smiled, feeling a deep sense of love and connection. "I feel the same way, Jake. We're in this together, and that makes all the difference."

Their commitment to supporting each other extended beyond the practical aspects of parenting. They made time for date nights, even if it meant simply sharing a quiet dinner at home after Emma was asleep. These moments of connection helped them maintain their relationship and reminded them of the love that had brought them together in the first place.

As they settled into their new roles, Sarah and Jake also recognized the importance of self-care. They encouraged each other to take breaks and pursue activities that brought them joy and relaxation. For Sarah, this meant taking long walks in the park, enjoying the fresh air and the simple pleasure of moving her body. For Jake, it meant finding time to play his guitar, losing himself in the music.

One Saturday, Jake encouraged Sarah to spend the afternoon with Emily, while he took care of Emma. "You deserve some time to yourself," he said, his eyes filled with love. "Go have fun with Emily. I've got everything under control here."

Sarah hesitated for a moment, but Jake's reassuring smile convinced her. "Okay, but call me if you need anything," she said, kissing Emma's forehead before heading out the door.

The afternoon with Emily was exactly what Sarah needed. They spent hours talking, shopping, and enjoying a leisurely lunch. For a few hours, Sarah felt like herself again, not just a new mother but also a friend, a woman with her own interests and identity.

When she returned home, she found Jake and Emma snuggled together on the couch, both of them fast asleep. The sight filled her heart with warmth and gratitude. She knew they were in this together, and their love and support for each other would see them through any challenge.

Building a support network wasn't just about seeking help from others; it was also about giving back. Sarah and Jake made a point to reach out to friends and family who were expecting or had recently become parents, offering their own experiences and support.

One evening, Sarah received a call from her friend Jessica, who was expecting her first baby. "I'm so nervous, Sarah," Jessica admitted. "What if I'm not ready for this?"

Sarah listened, offering words of encouragement and reassurance. "You're going to be an amazing mom, Jessica. And remember, you're not alone. We're all here to support you."

Jessica's gratitude was palpable. "Thank you, Sarah. It means so much to know I have friends like you."

As Sarah and Jake continued to navigate the ups and downs of parenthood, they felt a deep sense of gratitude for the support network they had built. Their journey had been filled with challenges, but they had faced them with the help of their family, friends, and community.

One evening, as they sat together in the nursery, watching Emma sleep, Sarah turned to Jake, her heart full. "I don't know what we would do without everyone's support," she said softly.

Jake nodded, his eyes reflecting the same gratitude. "We're lucky to have such amazing people in our lives. And we're lucky to have each other."

Their journey was far from over. There would be more sleepless nights, more moments of doubt and uncertainty. But there would also be more moments of joy, love, and connection. With their support network in place, Sarah and Jake felt ready to face whatever the future held, knowing they were not alone. They were surrounded by love and support, and that made all the difference.

As they embraced the joys and challenges of parenthood, Sarah and Jake knew that their support network was a vital part of their journey. It provided them with strength, comfort, and a sense of community. And as they looked ahead to the future, they felt a deep sense of gratitude for the people who had helped them along the way.

In the quiet moments, when the house was still and Emma was peacefully asleep, Sarah and Jake would often sit together, reflecting on the journey they had embarked upon. They knew that the road ahead would be filled with new challenges and experiences, but they also knew they had the love and support of their family, friends, and each other.

Together, they were building a life filled with love, laughter, and the promise of a bright future. And as they watched their daughter grow, they felt a profound sense of gratitude for the support network that had helped them become the family they were meant to be.

Chapter 12: The Birth Plan

As Sarah and Jake prepared for the arrival of their second child, they found themselves reflecting on their journey with Emma. Their experiences had taught them the importance of planning and being prepared, and they were determined to create a comprehensive birth plan this time around. The lessons they had learned from Emma's unexpected complications and early delivery were fresh in their minds, and they wanted to ensure that everything was in place for a smoother experience.

The decision to create a detailed birth plan was mutual. Both Sarah and Jake understood the value of being informed and proactive. They started by discussing their preferences and expectations for the birth process, knowing that clear communication and understanding were essential. They also consulted their healthcare provider, Dr. Roberts, to ensure their plan was realistic and medically sound.

One evening, after putting Emma to bed, Sarah and Jake sat at the kitchen table, their laptops open and a stack of pregnancy books nearby. "Okay," Jake began, "let's start with the basics. What are your preferences for labor and delivery?"

Sarah thought for a moment, then began to outline her thoughts. "I want to have as natural a birth as possible, but I'm open to pain relief options if needed. I also want you to be with me the whole time, and I'd prefer to avoid a C-section unless it's absolutely necessary."

Jake nodded, taking notes. "Got it. What about the setting? Do you want a hospital birth, or are you considering a birthing center or home birth?"

"I feel more comfortable in a hospital," Sarah replied. "Especially after what happened with Emma. I want to know that we have immediate access to medical care if anything goes wrong."

Jake agreed. "That makes sense. We'll make sure to choose a hospital that aligns with our preferences and has a good reputation for maternity care."

They spent the next few hours discussing various aspects of the birth plan, from the environment and pain management options to the presence of support people and post-birth care. They also researched different hospitals, looking for one that had a low C-section rate, a supportive staff, and positive reviews from other parents.

The following week, they scheduled a meeting with Dr. Roberts to discuss their birth plan in detail. They wanted to ensure that their preferences were feasible and that the medical team was aware of their wishes. Dr. Roberts was supportive and provided valuable insights, helping them refine their plan.

During the appointment, Dr. Roberts reviewed their birth plan. "This is a good start," she said, looking up from the document. "I appreciate that you've thought this through. It's important to be prepared, but also to remain flexible. Birth can be unpredictable, and sometimes we need to make adjustments for the safety of both mother and baby."

Sarah and Jake nodded, understanding the importance of flexibility. "We know things might not go exactly as planned," Sarah said. "But having a plan helps us feel more in control and prepared."

Dr. Roberts smiled. "That's the right attitude. Let's go through your preferences and see how we can support you."

They discussed pain management options, including the use of epidurals, nitrous oxide, and natural methods like breathing techniques and water immersion. Sarah expressed her desire to avoid an epidural if possible, but she appreciated knowing it was available if she needed it.

"We can also provide support with a birthing ball, massage, and different labor positions," Dr. Roberts explained. "Having a doula can be very helpful in managing pain naturally."

Sarah and Jake had already considered hiring a doula, someone who could provide continuous support during labor and delivery. They had met with a few doulas and were particularly impressed with a woman named Anna, who had a calming presence and extensive experience.

"We'd like to have Anna with us during the birth," Jake said. "She made a big difference in our comfort level when we met her."

Dr. Roberts nodded approvingly. "A doula can be a wonderful addition to your support team. I'll make a note of that in your file."

They also discussed the possibility of a water birth. The idea of laboring in a birthing pool appealed to Sarah, as she had heard it could help with pain relief and relaxation. Dr. Roberts informed them that the hospital had birthing tubs available and that they could include this option in their plan.

Another important aspect of their birth plan was the presence of family members. Sarah wanted her mother, Linda, to be there for emotional support, but she also wanted to ensure that the delivery room wasn't overcrowded.

"I think having my mom there will be really comforting," Sarah said. "But I don't want too many people in the room. It might get overwhelming."

Dr. Roberts reassured her. "We can limit the number of people in the delivery room. It's important for you to feel comfortable and supported."

As they continued to refine their birth plan, Sarah and Jake also considered the immediate postpartum period. They discussed their preferences for skin-to-skin contact, delayed cord clamping, and breastfeeding initiation.

"I want to have immediate skin-to-skin contact with the baby," Sarah said. "And I'd like to try breastfeeding as soon as possible."

Dr. Roberts agreed. "Skin-to-skin contact is very beneficial for both mother and baby. We'll make sure to facilitate that. And we have lactation consultants available to help you with breastfeeding."

Sarah felt a sense of relief knowing that her preferences were supported. The discussion with Dr. Roberts reassured her that they were on the right track and that their birth plan was realistic and achievable.

In the weeks that followed, Sarah and Jake continued to prepare for the birth. They attended childbirth classes, where they learned more about labor and delivery, pain management techniques, and newborn care. The classes provided them with practical knowledge and boosted their confidence.

One evening, after a particularly informative class, Sarah turned to Jake. "I feel so much more prepared this time around. I know we can't control everything, but at least we have a plan and the tools to handle whatever comes our way."

Jake squeezed her hand. "I feel the same way. We've got this, Sarah."

As they approached the final weeks of pregnancy, they focused on practical preparations as well. They packed their hospital bag, including items for comfort during labor, essentials for the baby, and snacks to keep their energy up. They also made arrangements for Emma's care while they were at the hospital, ensuring she would be well taken care of by her grandparents.

Sarah and Jake also took time to mentally and emotionally prepare for the birth. They practiced relaxation techniques, such as deep breathing and visualization, which they had learned in their childbirth classes. They also spent quiet moments together, talking about their hopes and dreams for their growing family.

One evening, as they sat on the porch, watching the sunset, Sarah leaned against Jake, feeling a sense of peace. "I'm so grateful for everything we've been through," she said softly. "It's made us stronger and brought us closer together."

Jake kissed her forehead. "I'm grateful too. We're ready for this, Sarah. No matter what happens, we'll face it together."

As the due date approached, Sarah and Jake felt a mixture of excitement and nervousness. They knew that the birth of their second child would be a unique and transformative experience, and they were determined to make it as positive as possible.

The day finally arrived. Sarah woke up early in the morning with mild contractions. She lay in bed for a moment, feeling the rhythm of her body and the anticipation building within her. She gently nudged Jake awake.

"I think it's time," she whispered.

Jake's eyes widened with a mixture of excitement and concern. "Are you sure?"

Sarah nodded, a calm determination in her eyes. "Yes. Let's get ready."

They moved with a practiced efficiency, gathering their hospital bag and calling Linda to come over and stay with Emma. Despite the early hour, Linda arrived quickly, her face filled with love and support.

"You've got this, sweetheart," Linda said, hugging Sarah tightly. "I'll take care of Emma. Just focus on bringing that little one into the world."

Sarah and Jake headed to the hospital, feeling a mix of nerves and excitement. The drive felt surreal, the streets quiet in the early morning light. As they arrived at the hospital, they were greeted by the friendly staff, who quickly got them settled into a birthing suite.

Anna, their doula, arrived shortly after, her presence immediately calming. She guided Sarah through breathing exercises and helped her find comfortable positions as the contractions intensified.

Hours passed, each contraction bringing them closer to meeting their new baby. Sarah focused on her breathing, drawing strength from Jake's presence and Anna's gentle encouragement. The birthing tub provided much-needed relief, the warm water soothing her aches and helping her relax.

Dr. Roberts checked in regularly, her calm and reassuring demeanor a constant source of comfort. She monitored the baby's progress and reassured Sarah and Jake that everything was going smoothly.

As the hours turned into the final stages of labor, Sarah's determination never wavered. She drew on the strength of her support network, knowing that she was surrounded by people who loved her and believed in her.

Finally, the moment arrived. With a final, powerful push, their baby entered the world. The room filled with the sound of newborn cries, a sound that brought tears of joy to Sarah's eyes. Dr. Roberts gently placed the baby on Sarah's chest, and she felt an overwhelming rush of love and relief.

"You did it, Sarah," Jake whispered, his voice filled with awe and pride.

Sarah looked down at their newborn, feeling a profound sense of connection and gratitude. "We did it," she replied, tears streaming down her face.

The next hours were a blur of joy and wonder. They held their baby close, marveling at the tiny fingers and toes, the soft skin, and the delicate features. They shared the news with their family, who rejoiced in the arrival of the newest member of their family.

As the sun rose on a new day, Sarah and Jake lay in the hospital bed, their baby nestled between them. They felt a deep sense of peace and fulfillment, knowing that they had brought their birth plan to life and welcomed their baby into the world with love and care.

Their journey was far from over, but in that moment, they felt a profound sense of accomplishment and joy. They were a family, bound together by love and the promise of a beautiful future.

As they drifted off to sleep, their baby snuggled close, Sarah and Jake knew that they were ready for whatever came next. They had faced the challenges of parenthood before, and they would continue to do so with love, strength, and the support of their family and friends.

The birth plan had been a guide, a source of reassurance and preparation, but it was their love and commitment to each other that had truly carried them through. And as they embarked on this new chapter of their lives, they knew that they were ready to face any challenge and embrace every joy, together.

Chapter 13: The Final Countdown

As Sarah and Jake approached the final weeks of pregnancy, the excitement and anticipation of their baby's arrival grew stronger each day. The nursery was ready, filled with soft pastel colors and baby essentials. Every corner of their home seemed to whisper the promise of new beginnings. Emma, too, was eagerly awaiting her sibling, often talking to Sarah's belly and asking questions about the baby.

The days were a mix of preparation and reflection. Sarah and Jake made sure they were as ready as possible, but also took time to savor these last moments before their family grew. They wanted to cherish the special times with Emma, understanding that their lives were about to change in beautiful, profound ways.

One sunny morning, Sarah woke up feeling a familiar tightening in her belly. It wasn't painful, just a gentle reminder that the baby was getting ready. She lay in bed for a few moments, rubbing her stomach and smiling at the thought of soon holding her newborn. Jake stirred beside her, and she gently nudged him awake.

"Morning," she whispered, her voice filled with warmth.

Jake opened his eyes, blinking away sleep. "Morning, love. How are you feeling?"

"Good," Sarah replied. "The baby's been moving a lot this morning. I think we're getting closer."

Jake's eyes lit up with excitement. "Really? How close do you think?"

"Hard to say," Sarah said, laughing softly. "But we should probably make sure everything is in order."

They spent the morning going over their checklist, ensuring that their hospital bags were packed and that all their plans were in place. Emma was particularly excited, helping Sarah pack a small bag with toys and books for the hospital.

"Is the baby coming today?" Emma asked, her eyes wide with curiosity.

"Maybe not today, sweetie," Sarah replied, smiling. "But very soon."

Emma nodded seriously, then patted Sarah's belly. "Okay, baby, we're ready for you."

As the days went by, the contractions became more frequent, but still irregular. Sarah felt a mix of anticipation and impatience, eager to meet her baby but also savoring the final days of pregnancy. She found comfort in her routine, spending time with Emma, taking walks with Jake, and practicing relaxation techniques they had learned in their childbirth classes.

One evening, as they sat on the porch watching the sunset, Jake turned to Sarah, his expression thoughtful. "Do you remember how we felt before Emma was born?"

Sarah nodded, leaning against him. "I was so nervous and excited. Everything felt so new and overwhelming."

Jake smiled. "It's amazing how far we've come. We're still nervous and excited, but in a different way. More prepared, I think."

Sarah agreed. "Definitely more prepared. And more confident. We know we can handle whatever comes our way."

The support from their family and friends was a constant source of comfort. Linda, Sarah's mother, called daily to check in, offering words of encouragement and advice. Jake's parents, Carol and Tom, also visited regularly, helping with household chores and spending time with Emma.

One afternoon, Carol and Tom arrived with a homemade casserole and a stack of baby clothes. "We thought you might appreciate a break from cooking," Carol said, setting the casserole on the kitchen counter.

"Thank you so much," Sarah said, giving them both a hug. "You have no idea how much we appreciate this."

Tom smiled, holding up a tiny onesie. "And we found these at a little shop downtown. Couldn't resist."

Sarah laughed, feeling a wave of gratitude. "They're adorable. Thank you."

As the final weeks turned into the final days, the anticipation reached its peak. Sarah's contractions became more regular and intense, signaling that labor was imminent. One night, she woke up with a sharp pain in her lower back, followed by a series of strong contractions.

She took a deep breath, trying to stay calm. "Jake," she whispered, gently shaking him awake. "I think it's time."

Jake's eyes flew open, instantly alert. "Really? Are you sure?"

Sarah nodded, gripping his hand. "Yes. The contractions are getting stronger and closer together."

Jake sprang into action, grabbing their hospital bags and calling Linda to come stay with Emma. Despite the urgency, he remained calm and focused, reassuring Sarah with his steady presence.

Linda arrived within minutes, her face filled with love and support. "You've got this, sweetheart," she said, hugging Sarah tightly. "I'll take care of Emma. Just focus on the baby."

Sarah nodded, feeling a surge of gratitude. "Thank you, Mom."

The drive to the hospital felt surreal, the streets quiet in the early morning darkness. Sarah focused on her breathing, leaning on Jake for support. When they arrived, they were greeted by the friendly staff, who quickly got them settled into a birthing suite.

Anna, their doula, arrived shortly after, her calming presence a welcome comfort. She guided Sarah through breathing exercises and helped her find comfortable positions as the contractions intensified. Dr. Roberts also checked in regularly, her reassuring demeanor a constant source of comfort.

As the hours passed, the contractions grew stronger and more frequent. Sarah focused on her breathing, drawing strength from Jake's presence and Anna's gentle encouragement. The birthing tub provided much-needed relief, the warm water soothing her aches and helping her relax.

Despite the intensity of labor, Sarah felt a sense of calm and determination. She knew that each contraction brought her closer to meeting her baby. Jake's constant support and the knowledge that they had prepared for this moment gave her the strength to keep going.

Finally, after hours of labor, Sarah felt an overwhelming urge to push. With Jake holding her hand and Anna encouraging her, she gave it her all. The room filled with the sounds of determination and support, everyone focused on welcoming the baby into the world.

With a final, powerful push, their baby entered the world. The room erupted in joyful cries as Dr. Roberts placed the baby on Sarah's chest. Sarah felt a rush of emotions, tears streaming down her face as she held her newborn close.

"You did it, Sarah," Jake whispered, his voice filled with awe and pride.

Sarah looked down at their baby, feeling a profound sense of connection and love. "We did it," she replied, her heart overflowing with joy.

The next hours were a blur of joy and wonder. They held their baby close, marveling at the tiny fingers and toes, the soft skin, and the delicate features. They shared the news with their family, who rejoiced in the arrival of the newest member of their family.

As the sun rose on a new day, Sarah and Jake lay in the hospital bed, their baby nestled between them. They felt a deep sense of peace and fulfillment, knowing that they had brought their birth plan to life and welcomed their baby into the world with love and care.

Their journey was far from over, but in that moment, they felt a profound sense of accomplishment and joy. They were a family, bound together by love and the promise of a beautiful future.

As they drifted off to sleep, their baby snuggled close, Sarah and Jake knew that they were ready for whatever came next. They had faced the challenges of parenthood before, and they would continue to do so with love, strength, and the support of their family and friends.

The final countdown had come to a beautiful conclusion, marking the beginning of a new chapter in their lives. And as they embraced their growing family, they knew that the journey ahead would be filled with love, laughter, and countless cherished moments.

Chapter 14: Labor and Delivery

The early morning air was crisp as Sarah and Jake drove to the hospital, their anticipation mounting with each passing minute. The contractions had grown stronger and more regular, signaling that labor was well underway. Sarah focused on her breathing, leaning on Jake's calm presence to steady her nerves.

Upon arriving at the hospital, they were quickly taken to the maternity ward. The bustling activity of the hospital was a stark contrast to the quiet tension in the car, but it was also comforting. Here, they were surrounded by professionals who would ensure the safety of both Sarah and their baby.

Dr. Roberts greeted them with a reassuring smile. "How are we doing, Sarah?" she asked, guiding them into a spacious, softly lit labor room.

Sarah managed a smile between contractions. "Ready as I'll ever be."

The room was equipped with all the necessary medical apparatus, but it also had a few personal touches to make it more comfortable: a birthing ball, soft lighting, and a chair for Jake. Anna, their doula, arrived shortly after, bringing with her a sense of calm and support.

"Let's start by getting you comfortable," Anna suggested, helping Sarah onto the birthing ball. "Remember your breathing techniques. You're doing great."

Jake held Sarah's hand, offering words of encouragement. The contractions were intense, but Sarah focused on the techniques they had practiced, finding a rhythm in her breathing. Anna guided her through different positions, each designed to help ease the pain and facilitate the labor process.

As the hours passed, the contractions grew stronger. Sarah leaned into the support of her team, drawing strength from Jake's steady presence and Anna's gentle guidance. Dr. Roberts monitored the baby's progress, reassuring them that everything was moving along smoothly.

"You're doing amazing, Sarah," Dr. Roberts said during one of her checks. "Everything looks good. Just keep breathing and take it one contraction at a time."

Sarah nodded, her face a mixture of determination and exhaustion. She focused on the end goal: meeting their baby. The pain was intense, but she knew it was a sign that her body was working hard to bring their child into the world.

The birthing tub, filled with warm water, provided much-needed relief. Sarah felt the tension in her body ease as she sank into the water, the buoyancy helping to support her weight and alleviate some of the pressure. Jake sat beside the tub, holding her hand and whispering words of encouragement.

"You're incredible, Sarah," he said softly. "I'm so proud of you."

Sarah leaned into his words, drawing strength from his unwavering support. The contractions continued, each one bringing them closer to the moment they had been waiting for. Anna helped Sarah find comfortable positions in the water, guiding her through the pain with gentle encouragement.

As the hours wore on, the pain became more intense, and Sarah felt a mixture of exhaustion and determination. She focused on her breathing, finding solace in the rhythm of the contractions. Each one was a step closer to meeting their baby, and that thought kept her going.

Dr. Roberts checked in frequently, her presence a constant source of reassurance. "You're doing great, Sarah. The baby is progressing well. Just keep listening to your body."

Sarah nodded, her grip on Jake's hand tightening with each contraction. The room felt like a sanctuary, filled with love and support. The pain was overwhelming at times, but she knew she was not alone. Her team was there, guiding her through each step of the process.

Finally, after hours of labor, Sarah felt an overwhelming urge to push. Dr. Roberts and Anna guided her through the transition, helping her find the right position. Sarah focused all her energy on the task at hand, drawing strength from within and from the support of her team.

Jake was by her side, his voice steady and reassuring. "You're almost there, Sarah. You're so strong. I love you."

With a final, powerful push, their baby entered the world. The room filled with the sound of newborn cries, a sound that brought tears of joy to Sarah's eyes. Dr. Roberts gently placed the baby on Sarah's chest, and she felt an overwhelming rush of love and relief.

"You did it, Sarah," Jake whispered, his voice filled with awe and pride.

Sarah looked down at their newborn, feeling a profound sense of connection and gratitude. "We did it," she replied, tears streaming down her face. The baby's tiny fingers curled around hers, and she felt a wave of love wash over her.

The next hours were a blur of joy and wonder. They held their baby close, marveling at the tiny fingers and toes, the soft skin, and the delicate features. They shared the news with their family, who rejoiced in the arrival of the newest member of their family.

As the sun rose on a new day, Sarah and Jake lay in the hospital bed, their baby nestled between them. They felt a deep sense of peace and fulfillment, knowing that they had brought their birth plan to life and welcomed their baby into the world with love and care.

The journey had been long and challenging, but it was worth every moment. They were a family, bound together by love and the promise of a beautiful future. As they drifted off to sleep, their baby snuggled close, Sarah and Jake knew that they were ready for whatever came next. They had faced the challenges of parenthood before, and they would continue to do so with love, strength, and the support of their family and friends.

The labor and delivery had been a test of their strength and resilience, but it had also been a testament to their love and commitment to each other. They had brought their baby into the world with grace and determination, and now they were ready to embrace the next chapter of their lives.

As they looked at their newborn, they felt a sense of awe and wonder. This tiny life they had created was a miracle, a symbol of their love and hope for the future. They knew that the journey ahead would be filled with challenges and joys, but they were ready to face it together, as a family.

The labor and delivery had been a transformative experience, one that had brought them closer and strengthened their bond. They had faced the pain and uncertainty with courage and determination, and now they were ready to embrace the joys and challenges of parenthood.

As they held their baby close, Sarah and Jake knew that they were ready for whatever came next. They had brought their baby into the world with love and care, and now they were ready to embark on the next chapter of their journey, together.

Chapter 15: Welcome to the World

The birth of their baby had been a profound and transformative experience for Sarah and Jake. As they lay in the hospital room with their newborn nestled between them, they felt a deep sense of accomplishment and joy. The tiny bundle in their arms was a symbol of their love and the culmination of their journey together.

The hospital room was quiet, the soft hum of medical equipment and the occasional footsteps of staff the only sounds breaking the silence. Sarah and Jake were wrapped in a cocoon of warmth and tenderness, their eyes never leaving their baby's delicate face. The newborn's tiny fingers curled around Sarah's finger, and the gentle rise and fall of the baby's chest was a soothing rhythm that filled the room with peace.

In the early hours of the morning, the sun began to cast a soft, golden light through the window. The hospital room was bathed in this warm glow, adding to the sense of tranquility and contentment. Sarah and Jake took turns holding their baby, marveling at every tiny detail. The baby's eyes, still adjusting to the world, blinked slowly as if trying to take in the new surroundings.

The arrival of their baby had brought a profound sense of wonder and connection. The initial moments of holding their child were filled with a sense of awe and gratitude. Every small movement, every tiny sound was a reminder of the miracle they had brought into the world.

As they looked at their baby, Sarah and Jake were overwhelmed by a wave of emotion. The joy of becoming parents again was coupled with a deep sense of responsibility and love. They were eager to learn every detail about their newborn, from the subtle cues and cries to the gentle ways of comforting and nurturing.

Throughout the day, the hospital staff came in to check on them, providing care and support. The pediatrician conducted a thorough examination, confirming that their baby was healthy and thriving. The nurses offered advice on feeding, diapering, and newborn care, answering any questions Sarah and Jake had with patience and professionalism.

The first feedings were a new experience for Sarah. With the support of a lactation consultant, she began to navigate the challenges of breastfeeding. The consultant provided tips and encouragement, helping Sarah to find comfortable positions and understand her baby's feeding patterns. The process was both rewarding and challenging, but Sarah was determined to give her baby the best start possible.

Jake was an attentive and supportive partner, assisting with diaper changes and comforting Sarah during the more challenging moments. His presence was a source of strength and reassurance, and together they began to find their rhythm as a family.

The hospital room was filled with the gentle sounds of their baby's soft cries and contented sighs. Sarah and Jake cherished these moments of bonding, feeling a deep sense of connection as they gazed at their child. They took turns singing softly and talking to their baby, their voices filled with love and affection.

In the afternoon, family members began to arrive, eager to meet the newest addition to the family. Linda, Sarah's mother, arrived first, her face lighting up with joy as she held her grandchild for the first time. "What a beautiful baby," she said, her eyes shining with tears of happiness.

Carol and Tom, Jake's parents, followed shortly after, their expressions a mixture of pride and excitement. They marveled at the tiny baby and offered their congratulations and support. The room was filled with a warm and loving energy as family members gathered to celebrate this special moment.

Emma, their eldest daughter, arrived with Linda, her eyes wide with curiosity and excitement. She approached the crib with a mix of awe and shyness. "Can I hold the baby, Mommy?" she asked softly.

Sarah smiled, carefully lifting the baby and handing her to Emma. "Of course, sweetie. Just be very gentle."

Emma held the baby with a sense of wonder, her little face glowing with pride and affection. "She's so tiny," Emma said, her voice filled with amazement. "I can't wait to play with her."

The family spent the afternoon visiting, sharing stories, and enjoying each other's company. The room was filled with laughter and joy as they celebrated the newest member of the family. Sarah and Jake felt a deep sense of gratitude for the love and support of their family and friends.

As the evening approached, the hospital room began to quiet down. The visits had ended, and the family was left alone to enjoy a few quiet moments together. Sarah and Jake reflected on the day, feeling a profound sense of fulfillment and joy.

With their baby sleeping peacefully in the crib, Sarah and Jake took a moment to embrace each other, their hearts full of love and gratitude. The journey to this point had been filled with challenges and uncertainties, but it had also been a journey of growth and discovery. They had faced the trials of labor and delivery with courage and strength, and now they were ready to embrace the joys of parenthood once again.

The hospital room, now calm and serene, felt like a sanctuary. The soft glow of the night lights created a peaceful ambiance, and the gentle rhythm of their baby's breathing was a soothing backdrop to their reflections.

As they held each other close, Sarah and Jake talked about their hopes and dreams for their family. They discussed the future, imagining the adventures and milestones that awaited them. Their conversations were filled with optimism and excitement as they looked forward to the journey of raising their new baby and continuing to nurture their growing family.

In the quiet of the hospital room, as the night settled in, Sarah and Jake felt a deep sense of peace. They knew that the days ahead would be filled with both challenges and joys, but they were ready to face them together. Their love for their new baby and each other was a source of strength and inspiration, guiding them as they embarked on this new chapter of their lives.

The birth of their baby had been a momentous occasion, one that had brought them closer and strengthened their bond. They had welcomed their child into the world with love and care, and now they were ready to embrace the future with hope and excitement.

As they settled into their new roles as parents, Sarah and Jake knew that they were surrounded by a supportive and loving family. They were grateful for the help and encouragement they had received, and they looked forward to creating many more cherished memories with their new baby and their growing family.

The journey of parenthood was just beginning, and Sarah and Jake were ready to embrace it with open hearts and a sense of adventure. They knew that the days ahead would be filled with both challenges and joys, but they were ready to face them together, united by their love and commitment to each other and their family.

With their baby peacefully sleeping beside them, Sarah and Jake felt a profound sense of fulfillment. They had welcomed their child into the world with love and care, and now they were ready to embark on the next chapter of their journey, together.

Chapter 16: Adjusting to Parenthood

The transition from hospital to home marked the beginning of a new chapter in Sarah and Jake's lives. With their baby safely nestled in the car seat, they made the journey from the hospital back to their home. The drive was a mixture of excitement and nervous anticipation. The streets seemed to pass by in slow motion as they reflected on the immense change that was about to unfold.

The house, previously a place of preparation and anticipation, now felt like a cozy haven ready to welcome their new family member. The nursery was set up with everything they needed: a crib, a changing table, and a small collection of toys and clothes. The sight of the room brought a sense of comfort and readiness, a reassuring sign that they were prepared for this new phase of their lives.

When they walked through the front door, the familiar surroundings felt both comforting and surreal. The quiet of the house was a stark contrast to the bustling activity of the hospital. Sarah and Jake exchanged glances, their expressions a mix of excitement and apprehension.

The first few days at home were a whirlwind of activity and adjustment. They found themselves quickly falling into the rhythm of new parenthood, navigating the demands of feeding, diapering, and soothing their baby. The constant cycle of feeding and sleeping left them feeling exhausted but profoundly fulfilled.

Sarah and Jake took turns caring for their baby during the night, trying to establish a routine that worked for everyone. Sleep deprivation became a familiar challenge, but they supported each other through it, finding solace in the quiet moments they shared while tending to their newborn.

One morning, as the sun filtered through the nursery window, Sarah and Jake found themselves sitting in the rocking chair, their baby peacefully sleeping in their arms. The stillness of the room was a welcome contrast to the chaos of the previous days. They took a moment to reflect on their journey, their hearts filled with gratitude and love.

"I can't believe how much has changed," Jake said softly, his voice filled with wonder. "It feels like just yesterday we were waiting for the baby to arrive."

Sarah nodded, her eyes filled with warmth. "It's amazing. It's also a lot of work. But it's worth every moment."

As the days turned into weeks, Sarah and Jake began to adjust to their new routine. They found a rhythm that worked for them, learning to balance the demands of parenthood with their own needs. They relied on each other for support, sharing the responsibilities and finding comfort in their partnership.

They also began to reach out to their support network, inviting family and friends to visit and offer their help. Linda, Sarah's mother, continued to be a constant source of support, offering practical advice and a listening ear. Jake's parents, Carol and Tom, were also a steady presence, helping with chores and providing much-needed encouragement.

The early days of parenthood were filled with small victories and challenges. Sarah and Jake celebrated each milestone, from the first time their baby smiled to the first successful feeding. They also faced moments of uncertainty, navigating the learning curve of parenting and adjusting to the demands of a newborn.

One evening, as they settled into their new routine, Sarah and Jake found themselves reflecting on their experiences. The challenges had been significant, but so had the rewards. They marveled at the strength they had found within themselves and each other, and they felt a deep sense of pride in their ability to navigate this new chapter of their lives.

"I never knew I could feel this way," Sarah said, her voice filled with emotion. "It's incredible how much love and joy a tiny person can bring into your life."

Jake smiled, reaching out to hold her hand. "I feel the same way. It's been a journey, but it's one I wouldn't trade for anything."

As the weeks went by, Sarah and Jake continued to adapt to their new roles. They found comfort in their routines and began to enjoy the simple pleasures of parenthood. The quiet moments spent with their baby became cherished rituals, and they learned to appreciate the small, everyday joys of family life.

Their baby grew and changed rapidly, and Sarah and Jake found themselves marveling at each new development. They captured each milestone with photographs and memories, cherishing the fleeting moments of infancy.

The support of their family and friends remained a constant source of strength. They continued to receive visits and offers of help, and the shared experiences and advice were invaluable. The community of support around them provided a sense of reassurance and comfort as they navigated the challenges of parenthood.

In the midst of the busyness of everyday life, Sarah and Jake made a conscious effort to nurture their relationship as a couple. They recognized the importance of maintaining their connection and finding moments of intimacy and relaxation. Whether it was a quiet dinner at home or a short walk together, they prioritized their relationship, knowing that it was the foundation of their family.

As they settled into their new routine, Sarah and Jake reflected on the journey of parenthood. They had faced challenges, but they had also experienced profound joy and fulfillment. The love they felt for their baby and each other was a guiding force, helping them navigate the ups and downs of their new reality.

The journey of adjusting to parenthood had been a transformative experience, one that had deepened their bond and strengthened their commitment to each other and their family. They had faced the challenges with courage and resilience, and they had embraced the joys with open hearts.

As they looked ahead, Sarah and Jake knew that the journey was far from over. Parenthood was a continuous process of growth and discovery, and they were ready to embrace it with enthusiasm and love. They were grateful for the support of their family and friends and excited for the future that lay ahead.

In the quiet moments of reflection, they felt a deep sense of gratitude for the opportunity to be parents once again. They knew that the journey of parenthood would continue to evolve, but they were confident in their ability to face it together, guided by their love and commitment to their growing family.

With each passing day, Sarah and Jake continued to embrace the joys and challenges of parenthood. They looked forward to the future with hope and excitement, knowing that their love and support for each other would carry them through the many adventures and milestones that awaited them.

The journey of adjusting to parenthood had been a beautiful and transformative experience, one that had enriched their lives and deepened their bond. As they embraced their new roles and the many joys of family life, they felt a profound sense of fulfillment and love.

Epilogue

The soft hum of the baby monitor filled the quiet of the house, its gentle sound a soothing reminder of the new life that had recently arrived. Sarah and Jake sat together on the sofa, their daughter sleeping peacefully in the nursery just down the hall. The exhaustion from the past few weeks was evident in their tired eyes, but it was a contented, fulfilled kind of weariness.

Their home, once a space of anticipation and preparation, now felt complete. The nursery, with its warm colors and carefully chosen decorations, was a testament to their journey and dreams. The small, intimate moments they had longed for were now their reality—feeding their baby, the soft lullabies, and the quiet, shared smiles.

As Jake reached over and took Sarah's hand, their fingers intertwined in a gesture of solidarity and love, they shared a look of deep satisfaction. The challenges of the past months had only strengthened their bond and deepened their appreciation for one another.

They were learning the rhythms of parenthood, navigating sleepless nights and the joys of new milestones with a sense of wonder and gratitude.

Their daughter, with her tiny fingers and gentle breaths, was a living symbol of their hopes and dreams.

In the stillness of the evening, surrounded by the gentle quiet of their home, Sarah and Jake felt a profound sense of peace. They were ready to embrace the future, knowing that every challenge would be met with love and every joy would be cherished. Their journey had only just begun, and they were eager to experience every moment together.

By

Gabreille Vicky

Growing Heartbeats Within

GABREILLE VICKY